# Reproductive Potential and Fertility Control

Edited by

**Catherine A. Niven RGN, BSc, PhD**
Reader in Psychology
Glasgow Caledonian University

and

**Anne Walker BSc, PhD**
Lecturer in Health Psychology
University of Leeds

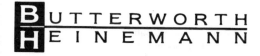

Butterworth-Heinemann Ltd
Linacre House, Jordan Hill, Oxford OX2 8DP

A member of the Reed Elsevier plc group

OXFORD LONDON BOSTON
MUNICH NEW DELHI SINGAPORE SYDNEY
TOKYO TORONTO WELLINGTON

First published 1996

© Butterworth-Heinemann Ltd 1996
© Chapter 10 Lorraine Sherr

**British Library Cataloguing in Publication Data**

A catalogue record for this book is available from the British Library

ISBN 0 7506 2249 0

**Library of Congress Cataloguing in Publication Data**

A catalogue record for this book is available from the Library of Congress

Typeset by EJS Chemical Composition, Midsomer Norton, Bath
Printed and bound in Great Britain by Hartnolls Ltd, Bodmin, Cornwall

# Contents

# Series preface

Sex, gender, adolescence, menstruation, pregnancy, childbirth, parenthood – these experiences are linked by their relationship to human reproduction. Reproductive experiences and behaviours can be divided into four broad categories. First, there are those concerned with the activity of reproduction: pregnancy and childbirth, for instance. Second are those to do with the potential for reproduction: puberty, menstruation and the menopause, for example. Going through puberty or having menstrual periods does not in itself constitute reproduction, but people who do not experience these things usually are not able to experience active reproduction either. What might be considered the prototypical reproductive activity, heterosexual sexual intercourse, does not fit neatly into either of these categories. In the late twentieth century, and perhaps for many centuries, only a minority of sexual acts are concerned with reproduction. The creation of another human being is only one of the many reasons for engaging in sexual activity of whatever type, so sex might be better considered as an activity with reproductive potential, rather than a reproductive act. A third category of activities and experiences are those concerned with fertility control: the things we do and decisions we make to control whether or not we have children. A fourth category is concerned with the consequences of reproductive activity: prenatal development, parenthood and parent–child relationships. These four elements of reproduction form a large part of many people's lives.

Reproduction is fundamental to human life. If we were all to decide tomorrow not to reproduce, then there would simply be no more people. How often we reproduce has economic and social implications for all areas of a society. The effects of the post-war 'baby boom' on education policy, employment possibilities and the care of older people can be clearly seen in our own society, for example. On a more global scale, the human population explosion has devastating environmental effects and significant qualitative costs for those humans who are produced, in terms of inadequacy of resources. Most governments attempt to control the reproductive activity of their people – either discouraging or limiting reproduction in a variety of ways, or promoting reproduction for religious or political reasons (Fathalla, 1992). Restrictive methods of control may range from the provision of family planning services and the discouragement of parenthood outside marriage to enforced sterilization programmes. Governments may encourage (or enforce) parenthood by not providing contraceptive information and/or access to abortion, by not educating women or encouraging women to be economically independent (hence promoting motherhood as the only choice). Clearly, reproduction is important for societies.

Reproduction is also a concern for individuals. Most people will have children at some time in their lives and are concerned about when to conceive children and how many children to have. Individuals, like governments, may be influenced by political, religious or economic factors in the desire to have children or remain child-free. Other more individual factors are involved though, such as a sense of identity as a parent, a need for 'immortality', pressure from potential grandparents, a desire to consolidate a relationship or a wish to be closely involved with a child from its earliest moments (see Walker and McNeill, 1991). Our society clearly sees the ability and desire to have children as 'normal' – writers in newspapers and magazines express sympathy for people who are unable to have children, and much money is spent on technologies to assist conception for the involuntarily childless. Choosing to remain child-free, by contrast, is less likely to be viewed positively, and women especially who decide not to have children may be seen as 'selfish' or 'unnatural' (Matlin, 1993).

Societies and cultures have not only controlled how many children people may have, but also the circumstances in which children may be conceived (e.g. only within marriage) and in which they are born (e.g. in hospital). In the late twentieth century control of conception has extended from the ability to prevent pregnancy (which has always been practised to some extent), to the ability, through technology, to enable conception in circumstances which would previously have prevented it. At present, the technology is far from perfect and many people who attempt to conceive using the new reproductive technologies are disappointed. However, the capacity for control both of conception and of gestation are present, with alarming moral and ethical implications, especially for women (Rowland, 1992; Chadwick, 1992).

Pictures of parents holding a longed-for baby whose conception was only possible through modern technology are emotive and heart-warming. Few of us could fail to be moved by them. They imply though that reproduction is a purely mechanical process, involving only the chance, or planned, meeting of sperm and egg. Of course, the physiological and mechanical processes involved in becoming pregnant, sustaining pregnancy and giving birth are important if we want to understand human reproduction. But as we have seen, reproduction has meaning both for individual men and women, and for society. Reproduction is not just a physical event. It also has psychological and social implications.

So, what is the 'psychology of reproduction'? From its earliest beginnings, psychologists have concerned themselves with some aspects of the reproductive process. Heterosexual sex and the development of gender identity have been of particular interest to researchers. Child development, both before and after birth, has also attracted attention. Few attempts have been made, however, to draw this research together as a coherent discipline. The establishment of the Society for Reproductive and Infant Psychology (SRIP) in the early 1980s, and its journal, the *Journal of Reproductive and Infant Psychology* (JRIP) in 1983, acknowledged the growth of psychological research in areas relating to reproduction, and the likely further growth in these areas resulting from the development of 'new reproductive technologies'. In the first editorial of the journal, Christopher Macy outlines the scope of reproductive and infant psychology as follows:

pregnancy and infancy ... might be regarded as central concerns within the field of reproduction .... But in order to understand women's experience of pregnancy we need to understand why women become pregnant .... We must look at the social value systems surrounding childbearing and childrearing, and equally at the psychological parameters associated with childlessness and infertility .... We take the view that psychological aspects of contraception and termination also fall squarely in our field as do many aspects of the psychology of women.

We would add to this by suggesting that many aspects of the 'psychology of men' fall into the remit of reproductive psychology too. The cultural tendency to see reproduction as 'women's work' has resulted in a neglect of men's experiences of puberty, fertility, contraception, sexuality, fatherhood and so on. The emphasis on women in this series of books should not be taken to imply that we consider reproduction only to be women's concern.

Reproductive issues have been approached from a variety of perspectives within psychology. The chief areas of interest have lain within clinical psychology and developmental psychology. Hence, the research which falls into the scope of reproductive psychology is dominated by 'problem-focused' studies and/or studies of infants and small children, rather than investigations of normative experiences. Not surprisingly, there is more to be said about repro- ductive activities and consequences than there is about reproductive potential and fertility control. Reproductive issues have attracted interest from a variety of other disciplines and epistemological movements too, which have influenced the approach of psychologists. The largest influence is that of the biomedical sciences. Since psychology has adopted similar research methods, and has often been concerned with similar research questions, biomedical themes have had a significant impact. This impact is shown in the concern of psychologists with psychiatric indices and labels of distress (e.g. post-natal depression) or with the psychological factors which predict distress, rather than understanding the experiences of people who are not distressed. Some psychologists have made important steps towards redressing this imbalance, however. For example, Myra Hunter's longitudinal studies of women going through the menopause (see Chapter 4 of this volume) have challenged the assumption from clinical studies that the menopause is necessarily a time of emotional turmoil and psychological dysfunction.

In addition to an emphasis on 'problems' such as post-natal depression, infertility, etc., the biomedical influence has also endorsed a positivist, hypothesis-testing approach within psychology. This approach usually requires measurement of experiences, and psychologists have played a role in developing a number of inventories and tools for quantifying distress or psychological state. Scores on such measures can be correlated with other factors in epidemiological surveys or used to evaluate interventions in treatment trials. Randomized controlled trials and measurement of experiences are clearly important in the appropriate context. However, the exclusivity of this approach in psychology has been criticized (e.g. Hollway, 1989; Potter and Wetherell, 1987). The emphasis on the use of existing measures can reduce the sensitivity of research to the specific experiences of participants in a particular study, and assumes that the quantification of experiences such as depression, joy, anxiety or pain is meaningful as well as functional. For these reasons, many researchers are turning towards qualitative or postmodernist approaches within psychology. In addition, a hypothesis-testing approach can encourage reductionism, that is the tendency to see the factor evaluated as the only important one. For example, if we test the hypothesis that anxiety management techniques reduce the intensity of pain during labour, and find them to be effective, then we (or others) may be tempted to infer that anxiety is the only important factor in labour pain. Clearly in this case that is a ridiculous conclusion. In other circumstances, though, the involvement of multiple factors may not be so apparent. The inadequacy of single-factor biomedical models to explain many modern health-related experiences has resulted in the development of biopsychosocial approaches to health and illness (e.g. Engel, 1977) and the birth of the new sub-discipline of health psychology. A biopsychosocial influence can be seen clearly in many of the chapters of this series, with reproductive psychologists avoiding reductionism by explicitly placing their work within a multi-factored framework (e.g. Ussher, 1992; Hunter, 1994). The influence of the biomedical approach and its emphasis on problems, quantification and reductionism will also be seen throughout this series.

A second influence is feminism and feminist theory. As we have already said, reproduction has historically been seen as the defining characteristic of womankind. The view of woman as a womb-container has had profound implications as many feminist writers have pointed out (e.g. Martin, 1989; Ussher, 1989). To attribute experiences such as premenstrual syndrome, postnatal depression, depression in middle age, emotionality in pregnancy, and so on, simply to the biological or psychological consequences of the female reproductive system is to ignore the effects of a patriarchal culture on women. Many feminist writers have described the inherent gender bias in modern societies which influences women's positions within heterosexual relationships, our earning capacity and the expectations held about the unpaid work we will do (e.g. Oakley, 1993). Women on average are poorer than men, whether employed or not. Women are more likely to be the recipients of domestic violence and sexual abuse. Women are more likely to care for children, ageing relatives or other dependent family members. In these circumstances it is at best misogynist to attribute distress solely to biological circumstances, or to attempt to adapt women's biology to enable us to cope with intolerable situations. So, feminist critiques are demanding the contextualization of women's reproductive experiences. A further impact of feminism in social science has been the questioning of power relationships within the research process and the critique of science itself as a patriarchal institution (see Harding, 1991). Medicine has been deconstructed as an instrument of social control – especially of women (see Ehrenreich and English, 1978; Showalter, 1987). Psychology too can be a powerful social control mechanism. The implications of this critique for the processes of doing research and reporting findings are far reaching. The interpretation of research as a political activity raises questions about who is doing the research, why they are doing it, who is paying for it and what the perceived benefits are. Many feminists are struggling to develop research methodologies which do not reinforce the imbalance of power between 'researcher' and 'researched', and which offer benefits for research participants in terms of empowerment, for example (see Neilson, 1990). These approaches have as yet had little influence on mainstream psychology, but the concern of reproductive psychology with the psychology of women means that they are having more of an impact here.

The purpose of this series of three books is to bring together the disparate strands of research and theory which can be called reproductive psychology. In our own work with undergraduate psychology, nursing and midwifery students, we have often felt the need for a single source of reference which could allow students to see the breadth and scope of psychological approaches to human reproduction. Our original intention was to bring these together in a single volume. The number of topics to be covered and the vigour of current research activity surprised us though, and we soon realized that a single volume would be inadequate to encompass it all. So, we have solicited contributions from currently active researchers for a three-volume series. The subject matter of each volume reflects the categories within reproductive psychology which we outlined at the beginning of this introduction. The first volume is concerned with reproductive potential and fertility control, the second with reproductive activity – conception, pregnancy and birth – and the third with the consequences of reproduction – early development, parenting and so on. There is no particular beginning or end to this series, although we have arranged the contributions in what seems to us to be a logical order. The circularity of human reproduction is apparent though; once the child has been born then she or he begins the process of gender identity and the development of their own reproductive potential, and so on. Like the seasons of the year, reproduction has no particular beginning or end. It is a continuous process, influencing all of our lives whether we are repro-ductively active or not. We hope that, like us, you will find the psychology of human reproduction, despite its inadequacies and omissions, a fascinating topic and that you will learn something of personal as well as academic interest from these books.

Catherine A. Niven
Anne Walker
1995

# References

Chadwick, R. (ed.) (1992). *Ethics, Reproduction and Genetic Control*. Revised edn. London: Routledge.

Ehrenreich, B. and English, D. (1978). *For Her Own Good: A Hundred Years of Experts' Advice to Women*. New York: Anchor Doubleday.

Engel, G. L. (1977) The need for a new medical model. *Science*, **196**, 129–36.

Fathalla, M. F. (1992). Society and reproductive life. In *Reproductive Life: Advances in Psychosomatic Obstetrics and Gynaecology* (K. Wijma and B. von Schoultz, eds) Carnforth: Parthenon.

Harding, S. (1991). *Whose Science? Whose Knowledge?* Milton Keynes: Open University Press.

Hollway, W. (1989). *Subjectivity and Method in Psychology: Gender, Meaning and Science*. London: Sage.

Hunter, M. (1994). *Counselling in Obstetrics and Gynaecology*. Leicester: BPS Books.

Macy, C. (1983). The Society for Reproductive and Infant Psychology: a statement of aims. *Journal of Reproductive and Infant Psychology*, **1** (1) 1–4.

Martin, E. (1989). *The Woman in the Body*. Milton Keynes: Open University Press.

Matlin, M. (1993). *The Psychology of Women*. 2nd edn. New York: Harcourt Brace Jovanovich.

Nielson, J. M. (ed.) (1990). *Feminist Research Methods*. Boulder, CO: Westview Press.

Oakley, A. (1993). *Essays on Women, Medicine and Health*. Edinburgh: Edinburgh University Press.

Potter, J. and Wetherell, M. (1987). *Discourse and Social Psychology*. London: Sage.
Rowland, R. (1992). *Living Laboratories: Women and Reproductive Technology*. London: Lime Tree.
Showalter, E. (1987). *The Female Malady*. London: Virago.
Ussher, J. (1989). *The Psychology of the Female Body*. London: Routledge.
Ussher, J. (1992). Research and theory related to female reproduction: Implications for clinical psychology. *British Journal of Clinical Psychology*, **31**, 129–51.
Walker, A. and McNeill, E. (eds) (1991). Family planning and reproductive decisions. *Journal of Reproductive and Infant Psychology*, Theme Issue, **9** (4).

# Preface

In the first volume of this three-volume series, we are concerned with the experiences and behaviours which are associated with reproductive potential and fertility control. Conception, pregnancy and birth are clearly the central features of the human reproductive process. They are not the beginning and end of reproduction though. Most humans spend only a small proportion of their lives actively engaged in reproduction. We are however capable of reproduction, and may be reminded of that by menstruation, puberty or the need to control our fertility. In this book, we cannot hope to cover every aspect of human reproductive potential and fertility control. The chapters which follow give a selection of the research in those areas which have been most interesting to psychologists. This is a biased selection in many ways. It is biased towards our own interests and concerns, and it is biased towards a white, middle-class and westernized perspective. There is much work to be done in exploring the diversity of reproductive experiences across divides of social class, religion, ethnic identity and sexual orientation, for instance. Psychology as a discipline has been slow to acknowledge that all people are not equal in opportunity or experience, and psychologists concerned with reproductive potential have not been exemplary in this regard.

The authors of these chapters adopt a variety of epistemological, substantive and methodological perspectives within social science. Some are clinical psychologists, others are academic researchers and teachers. Some adopt hypothesis-testing models in their own research work, others use social constructionist or post-modernist approaches. Some take an overtly feminist perspective, others do not. In this way, the chapters taken together provide a picture of the many influences on, and approaches within, reproductive psychology. They all provide up-to-date and evaluative reviews of their particular subject areas.

In the first four chapters, the concern is with aspects of reproductive potential which are quite separate from reproductive activity. In the first chapter, Gerda Siann considers gender and gender identity – the crucial psychosocial backdrop to human reproductive experience. In Chapter 2, Leo Hendry discusses the impact of puberty and sexual maturity within the complex and often lengthy process of adolescence. Chapters 3 and 4 are concerned with the experience of menstruation. Anne Walker in Chapter 3 asks whether women are psychologically disturbed by menstruation, while Myra Hunter in Chapter 4 explores the notion that the cessation of menstrual cycles at the menopause is psychologically deleterious.

Our reproductive organs are essentially 'private' in our culture, and at least partially hidden from immediate view. They are subject to disorders and dysfunctions as any system of the body is. In Chapters 5 and 6, the psychological aspects of examination and treatment of reproductive organs are considered. Susan Williams and Pauline Rafferty focus on psychological aspects of gynaecological procedures in Chapter 5, concentrating particularly on cervical screening ('smear' tests) and hysterectomy as examples. In Chapter 6, Kenneth Gannon considers the complementary medical specialism of andrology, and finds that psychological aspects of screening and treatment for testicular cancer and prostate conditions, for example, have been neglected in comparison with research into women's experiences.

Chapters 7, 8 and 9 are concerneed with fertility control – through contraception and elective abortion. In all of these chapters the authors are concerned with adults living in western cultures with freely-available contraceptive advice, making the point that these are concerns for all people and not just those living in the developing world. In Chapter 7, Elphis Christopher uses her experience as a family planning doctor in North London to put contraceptive use into the context of family planning while Paschal Sheeran, David White and Keith Phillips review the extensive psychological literature relating to contraceptive use by unmarried couples in Chapter 8. In Chapter 9, Anne Walker discusses the psychological predictors and consequences of pregnancy termination.

The final two chapters of the book investigate sexuality and sexual activity. These concerns lie on the border between reproductive potential and reproductive activity and have been the subject of intensive research and debate, particularly in recent years. We haven't tried to cover human sexuality comprehensively in this volume, but have included chapters from two authors whose work reflects particular current interests: the psychological aspects of HIV/AIDS, and female sexuality. In Chapter 10, Lorraine Sherr outlines the contribution that psychology has made to our understanding of 'risky' and 'safe' behaviours in the context of HIV/AIDS, while in Chapter 11, Jane Ussher criticizes the approach of traditional psychology to female sexuality and proposes new approaches for the future.

Throughout the book, the authors indicate the theoretical approaches taken to their subject as well as the findings which have accumulated, and advocate models of experience which integrate psychological factors with biological and social ones. We hope that these chapters will not only inform you about the state of research in reproductive psychology but also inspire you to adopt integrated biopsychosocial models of human behaviour in reproductive health-care practice and to conduct new research which will fill the many gaps which remain.

Catherine A. Niven
Anne Walker
1995

# Acknowledgements

The existence of these books owes a great deal to the Society for Reproductive and Infant Psychology. Most of the authors are members of SRIP, and it is through the activities of the Society that we have become aware of their work. At a more personal level, SRIP has enabled both of us to develop our research interests and discuss our research findings in a supportive and friendly atmosphere. Many SRIP members, past and present, have influenced our thinking and encouraged us to continue to work in this area. Particular thanks are due to the founder members of the Society, and editors of the *Journal of Reproductive and Infant Psychology*, whose vision and commitment have made the editing of these books possible.

Thanks are also due to the authors of these chapters who responded to our editorial demands with good humour and speed and to Susan Devlin and Deborah Humphries at Butterworth-Heinemann for their patience and efficiency.

# Contributors

**Elphis Christopher, MB, BS, DRCOG, DCH, MFFP, MIPM**
Elphis Christopher has been involved in family planning in a variety of settings –
clinics, young people's advisory work and domiciliary family planning, since
1966. She has been Senior Clinical Medical Officer for family planning in the
London Borough of Haringey since 1974. She runs psychosexual clinics at
University College Hospital, North Middlesex Hospital and Margaret Pyke
Centre. She has also done extensive sex education work in schools and youth
clubs for many years. She is the author of *Sexuality and Birth Control in
Community Work* (1987). She has also trained as a Jungian Psychotherapist, with
the British Association of Psychotherapists.

**Kenneth Gannon, BA, PhD**
Kenneth Gannon obtained his undergraduate and postgraduate degrees in
psychology at Trinity College, Dublin. He completed a training in clinical
psychology in Ireland before moving to London where he held post-doctoral
research fellowships at St Mary's Hospital Medical School and University
College London. He carried out research into the pelvic pain syndrome, recurrent
miscarriage and avoidable accidents in medicine. He is currently a senior
lecturer in behavioural science in the Royal London Hospital Medical College
where he teaches students of occupational therapy and medicine. He is carrying
out research into the psychological aspects of male infertility.

**Leo B. Hendry, MSc, MEd, PhD, FBPS, CPsychol**
Leo Hendry is Professor of Education at the University of Aberdeen. He has
published over eighty research journal articles and authored or co-authored
twelve books on adolescence, including *The Nature of Adolescence* (1990),
*Young People's Leisure and Lifestyles* (1993) and *Educating for Health: School
and Community Approaches with Adolescents* (1995). He has been involved in a
number of nationally funded research projects including a seven-year longitudinal study of the lifestyle development of 10,000 British adolescents: *Working
with Young People on Drugs Misuse and HIV/AIDS, The Benefits of Youth Work*
and *Young People's Perceptions of Health*. He has also contributed to various
edited books on young people in British society including *Unemployment:
Personal and Social Consequences, Youth Policy in the 1990s* and *Fit for Life?*
He has been a guest professor at several North American and European
universities, and is at present carrying out a study of adolescents and mentoring
for the Johann Jacobs Foundation.

## Myra S. Hunter, PhD, CPsychol, AFBPS
Myra Hunter is a clinical psychologist and senior research fellow/senior lecturer at Guy's Medical School, where she is co-ordinating research on menopause and midlife in primary care settings. She also works at University College London Hospital and Whittington Hospital where she is joint Head of Clinical Health Psychology Services, as well as managing the clinical psychology services to women's health. She is Clinical Director of the Women's Health Research Unit at University College London. Publications include *Counselling in Obstetrics and Gynaecology* (BPS) and *Time of Her Life* (Penguin/BBC).

## Pauline Rafferty, MA, PhD
Pauline Rafferty has obtained a PhD in the psychological aspects of gynaecological surgery and will shortly be undertaking a clinical psychology training course at the University of Edinburgh. She is currently teaching 'Introduction to Abnormal Psychology' at the Simon Fraser University in Vancouver, Canada.

## Keith Phillips, MA, PhD, AFBPs, CPsychol
Keith Phillips graduated from the University of Cambridge and completed his doctorate at the University of Hull, where he was then employed as a post-doctoral research fellow before appointment to a lectureship in psychology at the University of East London. He was Head of the Department of Psychology at UEL from 1989 to 1993, after which he was appointed to his current post as Professor and Head of The School of Social and Policy Sciences at the University of Manchester. He has published widely in the fields of psycho-physiology and health psychology.

## Gerda Siann, BSc, MSc, PhD, FBPS
Gerda Siann is Professor of Psychology at Glasgow Caledonian University. She is the author of numerous articles in the field of social psychology, and three books: *Educational Psychology in a Changing World*, (Allen & Unwin, 1980) (2nd edition Unwin-Hyman, 1988); *Accounting for Aggression*, (Allen & Unwin 1985) and *Gender, Sex and Sexuality: Contemporary Psychological Perspectives*, (Taylor and Francis, 1994).

## Paschal Sheeran
Paschal Sheeran is a lecturer in social psychology at the University of Sheffield. His research mainly concerns the self-regulation of behaviour. This has involved applications of motivational and volitional accounts of action to young people's contraceptive and HIV-preventive behaviours. He also researches the social psychology of identity, especially the impact of social structural position upon self-conception.

## Lorraine Sherr, BA Hons, Dip Clin Psych, BPS, PhD
Lorraine Sherr is a senior lecturer and Head of Health Psychology at the Royal Free Hospital School of Medicine. She is a consultant clinical psychologist working in AIDS and HIV and in obstetrics. She is joint editor of the *International Aids Care Journal* and founding editor of *Psychology Health and Medicine*. She has written a number of texts, including *HIV and AIDS in Mothers and Babies* (Blackwells), *The Psychology of Pregnancy and Childbirth* (Blackwells), *AIDS and the Heterosexual Population* (Harwood Academic),

*Grief and AIDS* (John Wiley) and *Death Dying and Bereavement* (Blackwell Scientific). She holds the current Chair of the British Psychological Society Special Interest Group on AIDS and is involved with a number of European initiatives on AIDS.

### Jane M. Ussher, BA, CPsychol, PhD

Jane Ussher is a lecturer in the psychology department, University College London, and Director of the Women's Health Research Unit at UCL. Her previous books include *The Psychology of the Female Body, Women's Madness: Misogyny or Mental Illness* and *Gender Issues in Clinical Psychology, The Psychology of Women's Health and Health Care* (both with Paula Nicolson), *Psychological Perspectives on Sexual Problems* (with Christine Baker). Her current research is on premenstrual syndrome, the long-term effect of child sexual abuse, and female sexuality.

### Anne Walker, BSc, PhD

Anne Walker is a lecturer in health psychology at Leeds University. She has been involved with menstrual cycle and premenstrual syndromes research for several years, recently expanding her interests to other areas of women's reproductive health. She is joint editor, with David Messer, of the *Journal of Reproductive and Infant Psychology*.

### David White, BSc, PhD

David White is Professor of Psychology at Staffordshire University. He was previously the Head of the AIDS Research Unit at the University of East London. He has published in the areas of health psychology and development psychology. His recent research activities include the development and evaluation of an intervention for the improved sexual health of injecting drug users.

### Susan Williams, MSc, SRN, SCM, HVCert

Susan Williams' main area of research is women's health medicine. Previous projects include *A Consumer View of Epidural; Analgesia* and *Alternative Forms of Antenatal Care*. She was awarded the Mary Thomson Research Fellowship in 1989 and has produced a consumer-led information and support package for women with abnormal cervical smears. She is now working at Greater Glasgow Health Board and in the Department of Nursing and Community Health, Glasgow Caledonian University, where she is currently looking into how health information material is being used by family doctors and practice nurses.

# 1

# Gender and gender identity

## Gerda Siann

The first four chapters of this book are concerned with normal aspects of reproductive potential. By this we mean the psychosocial experiences which are associated with the possibility of reproduction, rather than the activity of reproduction. Perhaps the most basic of these is our existence and identification as male or female. Human reproduction requires contributions from both male and female. This necessity has been inferred to mean that male and female are simple and biologically determined dichotomous categories, controlling not only whether we produce sperm or ova, but also our behaviour and psychological experiences – the 'mamawawa' or men-are-men-and-women-are-women attitude. In this first chapter, Gerda Siann asks whether our manliness or womanliness is solely determined by biology and explores the meaning of the terms sex and gender. How do we come to think of ourselves as male or female? Are some people androgynous? How can we explain the experiences of people who feel themselves to be trapped in the wrong sex body?

## Introduction

Public and media interest in gender is burgeoning. Sometimes it seems that no issue of a newspaper or magazine and no day's viewing on television is complete without reference to issues concerned with our identity as women or men, as 'feminine' or 'masculine'. The strength of this contemporary interest in gender emerges, I would argue, from social change in three areas. In the first place, economic pressures have increasingly eroded the distinction between male and female social roles. At its simplest, more women work outside the home than formerly and, relative to the past, fewer men do (Roberts, 1992; Moore, 1994). It is no longer unusual for men to care for children nor for women to head family groups. In the second place there is an increasing acceptance that sexual inequalities in educational and vocational opportunities are insupportable and this acceptance is now enshrined in legislation which outlaws sexual discrimination in law, in schools, colleges and universities and in the workplace (EOC, 1992).

Finally, increasing openness in the media about one of the most central aspects of our lives – our sexuality – has forced most people to think critically about their notions of masculinity and femininity (James and King, 1992). Prime-time television series such as *Brookside* feature lesbian and gay characters and documentaries frequently investigate issues such as transsexuality, cross-dressing and transvestism. In addition media exposure of celebrities like Madonna, Barry Humphreys in his incarnation as Dame Edna Everidge, Julian Clary and Sinead O'Conner has created in the general public a blurring of the certainties of earlier years which took for granted that men are 'masculine' and women are 'feminine' (MacDonald, 1995).

The first section of this chapter briefly examines the terms referred to above: sex, gender, sexuality, transvestism and transsexuality. Following this discussion contemporary psychological perspectives on sex and gender are outlined.

## Sex, gender and sexuality

At the moment of birth (and in recent times, often, even before birth), the first question asked about a healthy infant is: 'is it a girl or a boy?' (Siann, 1994). The answer to this question is, with very few exceptions, unambiguous, being dependent on biological characteristics, notably the external appearance of its genital organs, and for the remainder of the baby's life, again with extremely few exceptions, this categorization as either male or female will remain unproblematic (Unger and Crawford, 1992). Considerably more ambiguity, however, is attached to other interacting categorizations, such as gender and sexuality.

Social scientists have been particularly concerned with drawing a distinction between sex and gender (Hare-Mustin and Maracek, 1990). They have tended to do so in the following manner: *sex* is taken to refer to the biological differences between males and females and *gender* to the manner in which culture defines and constrains these differences. These constraints are seen as operating not only on the manner in which women, in general, live their lives compared to men, but also on the manner in which individuals view both themselves and others in terms of the female/male dichotomy. Obviously, then, gender and the two descriptors associated with it – feminine and masculine – are neither fixed nor immutable depending as they do on cultural variables. Not only are there differences between the kinds of behaviour expected from the sexes in different cultures; within cultures, these expectations have differed over time. In addition, the extent to which a culture constrains sexual differences in behaviour also varies considerably. For in hunting and gathering societies, such as the !Kung in Southern Africa there are minimal sex differences in social roles with both sexes caring for the young and taking responsibility for gathering food; in contrast 'the frail corseted Victorian lady in England' not only played a very different role from her spouse but was also regarded as very dissimilar in temperament and capabilities (Williams, 1987).

It is only relatively recently, however, that the majority of psychology texts have explicitly acknowledged that gender categorizations are relative rather than absolute and it is only even more recently that such texts have explicitly examined the extent to which biological sex determines sexuality (Caplan, 1987). Indeed consideration of aspects of sexuality other than those associated with heterosexuality received little attention in such texts until the last two decades. It is now, however, explicitly acknowledged in most psychology texts that sexual preferences and sexual orientation are not dependent only on biological sex. Consequently there is now more discussion of both the *practice* of homo- and bisexuality as well as discussion of issues surrounding the notion of sexual *orientation*. Thus the terms homosexual and lesbian are currently taken to refer to individuals who are not only sexually attracted to members of the same sex but who *identify* with other members of their own sex who feel the same way. The term bisexual is used to describe individuals of either sex who feel erotic attachments to members of both sexes although some researchers and clinicians maintain that there is no such thing as a 'true' bisexual because individuals who profess to be bisexual are really basically hetero- or homosexual (Unger and Crawford, 1992). The term, *transvestism* has been more recently superseded by 'cross-dressing' (Garber, 1993) and is used to describe the practice of dressing in the clothes, and taking on the appearance, of members of the other sex. Cross-dressing has a long tradition in the theatre, partially rooted in the fact that until the eighteenth century women were seldom permitted to appear on the stage. In addition, probably because of the restricted social roles open to women, there are many documented instances of women who lived out their lives as men, for example Deborah Sampson, an eighteenth-century woman who served in the US army, was decorated and only discovered to be a woman when hospitalized (Williams, 1987).

Recently cross-dressing has attracted a great deal of media attention which has focused not only on the cross-dressing of drag artistes and male homosexuals who work as prostitutes but also on individuals, the majority of whom are males, who cross-dress at home and sometimes in social groups with other cross-dressers. While it is widely believed that transvestism is linked to homo- or bisexuality, research indicates that the majority of cross-dressers are heterosexual (Ruse, 1988).

Most cross-dressers, irrespective of their sexuality whether homo-, bi- or heterosexual, do not question their biological sex. However a minority, who differ in no way *physically* from others of their sex, feel convinced that they are trapped in a body of the wrong sex. These individuals, who are termed *transsexuals*, are frequently very keen to undergo extensive surgery and hormone treatment to remedy this. A well-known example is the journalist Jan (formerly James) Morris who has described how, from her earliest childhood, although her appearance was stereotypically male, she was unhappy with her identity as a boy. This unease culminated in an active desire physically to change her identity from male to female despite a successful career as a foreign correspondent and despite marriage and fatherhood (Morris, 1974).

It has been estimated that there are 30 000 transsexuals in the world and, concurrent with the recent proliferation of surgical treatment of transsexuals, a number of studies have been carried out on their psychological adjustment after surgery. The results of these studies are by no means consistent, in that while some have indicated overall positive outcomes after surgery others have indicated that after surgery some transsexuals appear less well psychologically adjusted than before (Unger and Crawford, 1992).

Such studies with their inconsistent outcomes do, however, emphasize the complexity of the relationship between sex, gender and sexuality and point to the inherent difficulties surrounding the relationship between biology and gender. Speculation about these relationships often crystallizes round the question: 'Is biology destiny?' and I will now consider responses to this question.

## Essentialist perspectives

The view that females and males are essentially different in nature, and that biology *is* destiny, has deep historic roots in both western and non-western cultures and permeates mythology, literature and philosophy in most cultures (Ussher, 1989). It is not surprising, then, to find such views (frequently termed 'essentialist'; Hare-Mustin and Maracek, 1990) reflected in certain approaches to the psychology of sex and gender, notably in two contrasting perspectives, biological determinism and psychoanalysis.

## Biological determinism

This viewpoint proposes a very direct link between sex and gender. Biological determinists argue that the certain and fundamental aspects of the nature of femininity and masculinity (or gender differences) are constant across all cultures and across all time periods because *in essence* biological differences between the sexes constrain the psychological functioning of the two sexes in different ways. Many (but by no means all) adherents of this viewpoint draw on evolutionary theory to argue that human society has evolved in such a way that men have the innate qualities and attributes of the hunter, whereas women's innate predispositions are towards attributes and qualities associated with domesticity.

Many biological determinists argue that 'sexual dimorphism' or the existence of two different forms of most species arose because it provides a mechanism for increasing diversity within species by providing two sets of genetic material out of which individual members of a species can be created (Williams, 1987).

In humans it is argued that hormonal differences between the sexes starting during pregnancy with the action of androgens in the case of male (XY) embryos and continuing throughout the life span, but notably during gestation and at puberty, constrain the psychological and in some cases the cognitive development of the two sexes in such a way that throughout all cultures and during all epochs men and women will differ in their psychological and cognitive functioning. Thus from the viewpoint of biological determinism, the nature of men and women or 'masculinity' and 'femininity' is characterized by certain invariant differences.

The differences cited normally fall into two categories. The first category is associated with *psychological attributes*. These are often cited by sociobiologists such as E. O. Wilson (1975) who assert that evolutionary forces constrain sex differences in such a way that men are by nature more adventurous, competitive and aggressive than women. Certain feminist theorists, such as Alice Rossi (1987), while concurring with sociobiologists that sex differences in psychological attributes characterize all cultures and epochs, emphasize a different set of psychological sex differences, arguing that women are by nature more sensitive and empathic than men because evolution has predisposed mothers to possess innate sensitivities to newborn babies. It should be noted, however, that recent anthropological studies focusing on gender have indicated that in a number of hunting and gathering societies there are minimal differences in the social roles of men and women and correspondingly minimal differences in the personal qualities and traits attributed to the sexes (Sanday and Goodenough, 1990).

The second set of sex differences cited by theorists working from within the tradition of biological determinism are associated with *cognitive* attributes. Thus Rushton (1992) argues that men's cranial capacity is bigger than women's because evolutionary pressure necessitated male superiority in the spatial skills demanded in hunting and finding their way back home and that it is in order to accommodate these skills that male brains are larger than female brains.

The evidence cited by biological determinists to support their position comes from six sources. First, studies of individuals who were exposed when *in utero* to high levels of sex hormones normally associated with the opposite sex, e.g. mothers of girls exposed to high levels of male hormones during pregnancy

(Ehrhardt and Meyer-Bahlberg, 1981). Second, studies of individuals with chromosomal abnormalities, e.g. men with the XYY chromosomal pattern (Witkin et al., 1976). Third, studies of individuals with hermaphroditic conditions (Unger and Crawford, 1992). Fourth, studies concerned with the link between the levels of male hormones like testosterone and levels of aggression (Siann, 1985). Fifth, studies concerned with the link between mood change in women and hormone levels (Ussher, 1989) and finally, studies concerned with similarities in brain function between brains of women and the brains of male homosexuals (Le Vay, 1993).

An excellent review of the biological determinist perspective can be found in Le Vay (1993) and a spirited attack on the perspective in Fausto-Sterling (1992).


## Psychoanalytic perspectives

Psychoanalysts starting with Freud have tended to argue that the nature of familial dynamics, predominantly in the third to fifth years of life, predisposes men and women, in general, to develop differing sets of psychological attributes and that so powerful is this predisposition that there are unambiguous and *essential* differences in male and female psychology. It is beyond the scope of this chapter to do more than describe one contemporary development of the psychoanalytic tradition which bears on the nature of gender development. This is the view put forward by Chodorow (1979) which has had a powerful influence on psychoanalysts working from a feminist perspective.

Nancy Chodorow retains in her work Freud's emphasis on the effect on gender differences of the experiences of infancy. In fact she traces these to a period before the Oedipal stage when, because the infant is small and helpless, it is totally reliant on its chief caretaker, whom Chodorow takes to be normally its mother. The child initially has great difficulty in differentiating itself from its mother but with growing physical and cognitive maturation begins to define itself in relation to its primary caretaker.

This process develops differently for boys and girls. Girls grow up with a sense of similarity to, and continuity with, their mothers while boys have to learn a different sense of gender identity and, because fathers are less often present than mothers, they have a more precarious sense of gender identity. In order to compensate for this they become more concerned than girls with knowing what is 'masculine' and what is 'feminine' and in drawing the boundaries between these attributes. Mothers contribute to these growing differences, according to Chodorow, because they have themselves been girls and consequently they experience their daughters as an extension of themselves but their sons as 'male opposites'. In this way they encourage girls to identify with them and boys to differentiate themselves from them.

Chodorow argues that these early gender differences in identity formation have important consequences for personality differences in later life. Girls emerge with a capacity for 'empathy' and a set of emotional needs which are tied to the desire for being connected to other human beings and which commit them to the destiny of nurturing others, notably their own children. Boys, on the other hand, who have learned to define masculinity as the opposite of femininity grow into men who devalue women and who believe in the superiority of whatever qualities they define as masculine.

Thus, according to Chodorow, each generation reproduces the traditional sex differences of caring empathic women and rational and achieving men not because of their biology but because masculine–feminine differences are continually 'reproduced' in the dynamics of early family life. Thus, while rejecting Freud's emphasis on the importance of the Oedipal stage and penis envy, she accepts his basic argument that later personality development, and consequent sex differences, depend crucially on the earliest years of life and their influence on unconscious processes. Chodorow's influence can be traced in the work of a number of contemporary women therapists who are concerned particularly with working with women.

As is well known, theorists working within the psychoanalytic tradition base their theories on clinical experience. Hence early psychoanalysts like Freud as well as contemporary ones like Chodorow cite case histories rather than empirical studies in support of their theories.

# Socialization perspectives

In the consideration of gender issues psychology has drawn very minimally on either of the two perspectives outlined above. Rather, it has been influenced by the behaviourist, social learning and latterly cognitive paradigms and has tended to endorse the view that biology does not determine gendered behaviour and to consider gender within the context of socialization.

From this perspective men and women are seen to differ mainly because of differences in the manner in which their particular society shapes and moulds their behaviour, attitudes and values.

## Behaviourism and social learning

Behaviourists explain gender differences (or sex differences) by the general principle that boys are rewarded for masculine behaviour and girls for feminine. In support of these claims, behaviourists pointed to the many instances of parents and other adults openly approving and rewarding particular and different behaviours for boys and girls (Unger and Crawford, 1992).

Early behaviourists tended to emphasize the importance of the contingent effect of particular acts. Thus they saw children's behaviour as shaped by direct rewards, praise, punishment or disapproval. Later workers in the tradition, however, like the social learning theorist Albert Bandura developed the notions of latent learning from social situations and modelling (Bandura and Walters, 1963). They pointed out that a parent does not need consciously to approve or disapprove of particular behaviour or indeed intend to shape different behaviours in boys and girls. The learning process may be latent and far less deliberate because of the child's propensity to copy and imitate the actions of others and to 'model' their own behaviour on the observed behaviour of others with whom they 'identify'.

But if we do accept that children 'learn' how to behave by imitation and modelling, we are left with the question of whom they choose for models and why they make such choices. Social learning theorists, basing their claims on laboratory studies, argued that children tend to imitate the actions of, and model themselves on, those whom they perceive to be friendly, warm, attentive, powerful and similar to themselves (Bandura and Huston, 1961). If this were the case for gender development, social learning theorists would have to demonstrate that men and women are attractive role models for boys and girls respectively. Empirical studies, however, offer only inconsistent support for these claims. For example, a review of twenty laboratory studies in which children were presented with models of both sexes revealed little consistent tendency for preschool children to select same-sex models. When shown models who were displaying affection, aggression, toy choices, aesthetic preferences, and other activities, the children's choices were not apparently affected by the sex of those they chose to model (Maccoby and Jacklin, 1974). Further, while some studies do show parent–child similarities on certain dimensions of personality such as values and attitudes, they fail to show that these similarities are related to the sex of the parents (Williams, 1987). This lack of support for this central tenet of social learning approaches to gender combined with a general movement in mainstream psychology away from social learning approaches has led to an emphasis on the role of cognition in development, and this approach will be considered next.

## Cognitive developmental approaches

Cognitive perspectives on gender question the central tenet of the social learning approach to gender which is that the child is passively shaped by external contingencies. Instead cognitive theorists focus attention on the active manner in which children strive to make sense of their social environment

In their consideration of the child's active attempts to make sense of gender, cognitive developmental psychologists like Lawrence Kohlberg (1966) define three terms: gender identity, gender typing and sex role. The term *gender identity* refers to the psychological sense of oneself as female or male. The term *gender typing* refers to the process of developing traits and behaviours that mirror the views of one's society about what is appropriate for a male or female. The term *sex role* refers to the set of behaviours considered appropriate for females or males within a particular culture (Deaux, 1987). According to Kohlberg and his associates, gender identity and gender typing develop in a fixed manner and, in agreement with Piagetian theory (Piaget, 1954) in three discrete stages. The first stage is reached between two-and-a-half and three years when the child achieves gender identity. At this stage children can identify themselves correctly as a girl or boy and can also correctly identify the sex of others both in real life and from pictures. The second stage occurs when gender stability is reached (about age five). At this stage children realize that they will retain the same gender throughout life.

However, while children at this stage understand that their own gender won't change, they do not realize that the same applies to other people. According to Kohlberg and others, the child's understanding of gender is still very concrete and limited. It does not extend to understanding that changing outward gender attributes does not change gender. The third stage, gender constancy, only emerges at around seven years of age. This final change involves the deep understanding that if an adult were to change their physical appearance completely (as in the case of a drag artist), their gender would not change.

It is important to understand that Kohlberg and his associates believe that the child moves through these stages not, as the social learning theorists argue, because he or she is rewarded and moulded into sex-typed behaviour but because, having acquired gender identity, the child actively selects from the repertoire of social behaviour he or she is exposed to, those elements that are appropriate to his or her gender identity. Further, where social learning theorists see identification with the same sex adults or peers as causing sex typing, Kohlberg argues for the reverse – that is it is only after the child has achieved gender identity and has started gender typing him or herself, that he or she then identifies with same sex peers and adults.

Kohlberg would not deny that society can reinforce sex-typed behaviour but would claim that this is an additional source of sex typing rather than its prime vehicle.

Critiques of Kohlberg's views on gender development have tended to centre on its male bias in that he used the gender development of boys as the model for his theory, generalizing it to girls only later (Rohrbaugh, 1981). In addition to the relative weakness of Kohlberg's theory when it is applied to females, his approach has also been criticized by Bem (1983) amongst others, because it fails to ask why it is that sex is the major category by which children come to categorize themselves.

Finally it should be pointed out that research has not supported Kohlberg's claim that children become sex-typed only after achieving an understanding of gender constancy. On the contrary, as Unger and Crawford (1992) point out, empirical studies show that most children show a preference for gender-typed objects and activities by the age of three, before gender constancy is normally achieved.


## Moving beyond gender typing

### Androgyny

The next major development in the psychological study of gender to follow on from the cognitive developmental approach was related to the critique of mainstream psychology which was starting to emerge from the growing ranks of women psychologists in the 1970s and 1980s, when spokeswomen such as Mary Parlee (1985) and Carole Gilligan (1982) began to make explicit the largely male-centered nature of the discipline. They pointed out that theories had largely been constructed from the 'male-as-normative viewpoint' by male psychologists frequently using as 'subjects' samples of students who were predominately male. (Concurrently attention was also being drawn to the fact that most psychologists within the western world were also white and middle class; Siann and Ugwuegbu, 1988).

Pre-eminent among the women critics of mainstream psychological approaches to the psychology of gender was Sandra Bem, who began to explore the relevance to this area of the concept of 'androgyny'. The word androgyny combines the Greek roots andro (male) and gyn (female) to refer to a balance of both, and the underlying concept of androgyny as a blending of masculine and feminine attributes has a long history with roots in classical mythology, literature and religion. Thus to say a person is androgynous suggests that the individual concerned has attributes, physical, psychological or both, that do not reflect the prevalent separate sex typing of their culture. For example, in the mid 1970s David Bowie, and in the 1980s Annie Lennox and Grace Jones, presented physical personae that could be regarded as androgynous.

Bem pioneered a simple questionnaire: the Bem Sex Role Inventory (BSRI). According to her original formulations, scores on this inventory could be grouped into three categories: male-typed, female-typed and androgynous. Work using the BSRI suggested that individuals falling into the androgynous category functioned better and more flexibly than their more conventionally sex-typed peers (Spence, Helmreich and Stapp, 1975).

In the later 1980s methodological criticisms began to emerge both of the content of the BSRI scale and of its scoring. Further doubt began to be thrown on the empirical results linking androgyny with superior adjustment and mental health (Unger and Crawford, 1992). In addition, Bem herself began to reject the notion that there are independent variables such as masculinity and femininity and she, with many others, began to move towards an alternative formulation of the psychology of gender: gender schema theory.

## Gender schema theory

Gender schema theory contains some elements of both the cognitive and the social learning approaches to development. In accordance with social learning approaches, the theory acknowledges the framework of learning provided by the social world. In accordance with many cognitive approaches, it argues that young children construct cognitive 'schemas' to help them understand and come to terms with both the external world and their own internal representation of it.

The term schema refers to the mental structures children use to encode and process information. Basically schema theory suggests that schemas and scripts (the term 'script' is used by cognitive theorists to describe the child's understanding of a likely sequence of events) provide cognitive tools for thinking about the past, present and future. They are essentially networks of associations and general knowledge which aid thinking about and understanding not only the external world but also the internal one. Furthermore, they provide a set of flexible cognitive networks into which new experiences or information can be assimilated. Thus children will not only have schemas and scripts about referents in the social and physical environment, such as bedtime, going to visit the dentist, what a typical boy or girl is like and what a naughty child is like; they will also have schemas about themselves.

Applying schema theory to gender, Bem (1983) suggests first that sex typing is a gender schema that varies from culture to culture. Drawing from learning theory, she proposes that the cultural content of gender schema will undoubtedly be affected not only by what the society labels as appropriately masculine or feminine behaviour, but also by the extent to which the culture or subculture rewards or punishes adherence to such sex typing. Second, she proposes that self schemas (or the manner in which individuals think about themselves) are permeated to differing degrees by gender schema, both across individuals and, in the case of any particular individual, across time and social contexts.

In this way any particular individual growing up in a particular society will acquire knowledge and feelings both explicit and implicit about the gender typing of their own culture, subculture and domestic environment. This will give them a readiness to process and organize other schemas, including their own self schema, with reference to gender schemas. Some individuals will have fairly rigid gender schemas, closely related to cultural stereotypes which they will frequently, if not invariably, use as tools in order to organize and evaluate their own behaviour and to evaluate the behaviour of others. Such individuals would be regarded by Bem as 'strongly sex-typed'. Individuals with a less rigid gender schema which they relate less frequently and less strongly to themselves and others, Bem would regard as 'weakly sex-typed'.

Moving away from this theoretical base to a more *prescriptive* platform, Bem recommended that gender schemas should play a less important role in society than they do at present. She also proposed that we should encourage individuals to view themselves less through the lenses of gender schemas. Additionally she began to argue that the gender dichotomy has, until very recently, spelt out an inferior role for women and a superior role for men in most societies.

### The lenses of gender

In her recent work, Bem has expanded and developed her position in two ways, moving her focus from the individual to the cultural (Kitzinger, 1992). First, she has pointed out the extent to which gender as an heuristic for making sense of the world continues to dominate social and personal life. Second, she has emphasized the extent to which contemporary society continues to use gender as the pre-eminent criterion for segmenting and structuring social life. This stance brings her very close to social constructionist and post-modern psychologists whose views will be considered next.

## Social constructionist approaches

Social constructionist is a term that is used by American theorists who write about the psychology of gender from an overtly feminist perspective (Hare-Mustin and Maracek, 1990). This perspective suggests that gender operates at individual, interpersonal and cultural levels to structure people's lives. It challenges one of the key assumptions of mainstream approaches to psychology by contesting the traditional contention that psychologists can operate from a value-free and 'objective' stance. On the contrary, social constructionists argue that traditional approaches are neither value free nor objective. These approaches have been dominated by the presumptions (and frequently the biases) of middle class, white males. As evidence for these assertions they point to the work of psychologists like Lawrence Kohlberg whose theories were built on studies conducted with groups of subjects which were almost exclusively male.

Social constructionists also point out that in most societies, until very recently, males have dominated females. This has given males a power base from which male achievements have been overvalued and female achievements under-valued. For example, they point to the fact that while it has been frequently reported that women score higher than men on many tests of verbal ability and men score higher than women on many tests of mathematical ability, media attention is focused on the areas in which men do better than women, rather than the reverse (Fausto-Sterling, 1992).

Social constructionists argue that it is the dominant groups whose power and assumptions shape our social world. They also take into account that male dominance and power over females is frequently overlaid and complicated by social class and ethnic differences.

Evidence supporting social constructionist approaches can be found in many studies which indicate that identical behaviour carried out by men and women is frequently rated and appraised in different ways, for example when a female manager is perceived as 'bossy' but a male manager behaving identically is perceived as 'authoritative' (Siann, 1994; Unger and Crawford, 1992).

## Post-modern approaches

Recently a number of feminist psychologists, influenced by the French thinker Foucault (1979), have written about gender issues from what has been called a 'post-modernist' perspective.

In general the post-modernist movement in the social sciences disclaims the search for enduring, absolute and universal truths. Instead its protagonists argue that it is impossible to escape the bias of our own personal and cultural positions (Tong, 1989). In this way it echoes the social constructionist approach.

The post-modernist position, however, goes further than this. It not only argues that it is difficult, if not impossible, to agree about the 'objective' nature of the outside world, but it also maintains that our experience of our internal world is also, at its core, fragmentary and shifting. In essence, it denies that we have any stable and coherent internal 'self' – instead it argues that we continually change and 'position' ourselves. For example, a woman scientist may 'position' herself as a caring mother in conversations with a group of other young mothers, but as an ambitious scientist in conversation with a group of young scientists. This positioning is not only actively carried out; it is also in a sense forced on her by different social dynamics. Other people treat you differently depending on the social role you are perceived to be playing. In addition, according to Hollway (1989) we don't actively position ourselves all the time. In many instances our 'positioning' is unconscious and may only reveal itself when we take up different positions in our discussions and inter-actions with others.

A young man may, of course, also 'position' himself differently at different times. For example, as a loyal fan of a football club on a night out after a Cup Final on the one hand, and as a responsible young father when applying for a bank loan, on the other. But if he is white and middle class, because his social and gender groups are those dominant in society, he has to shift his position less. In general, according to those arguing for a post-modernist approach, multiplicity is less characteristic of dominant groups than of those with lesser social power. So, for example, 'multiplicity' of positioning is more charac-teristic of black groups than white.

In order to illustrate this point Hollway (1989) quotes Amina Mama on the differential social pressures operating on members of the ethnic minority and ethnic majority communities in the West:

> The capacity to occupy many social positions is true of many, if not all, black people who have lived in the West, in ways that are not necessarily so for

white people who have lived in Third World countries because of the historical status of expatriate communities as colonisers.

Thus, like the feminists working from social constructionist approaches, post-modern feminists emphasize the manner in which power and status imbalances between the sexes (or indeed between ethnic groups) contribute to differences in social behaviour between the sexes and between social groups.

The approaches to gender which have been considered in this section, i.e. those of Bem, social constructionists and post-modernists, offer little endorsement of the proposition that biology is destiny. Rather they frequently substantiate their arguments by pointing to studies, many of which are drawn from anthropological sources (Siann, 1994; Tavris and Wade, 1984) which indicate the extent to which cultural values permeate notions of gender and they explicitly draw attention to the manner in which the power imbalances between the sexes tend to favour 'masculine' rather than 'feminine' modes of behaviour.

## Conclusion

It is clear that the accounts that are currently offered of the development of gender vary greatly. Those accounts which have been termed 'essentialist' in this chapter tend to resonate with the intuitive feelings held by many people that there are pervasive and deep-seated differences in the basic nature of men and women. Such viewpoints often underpin articles, television programmes and films which argue that advances made by women in the social and economic fields bring with them inevitably negative consequences in that women are no longer committed to their true destiny, which is to nurture and care for others (Lyndon, 1992). Related to this perceived betrayal by women of their 'essential nature' is a perceived threat to the status and power of men because many women are now in charge of their own personal and economic destiny (Thomas, 1993). Views such as these tend to be articulated more frequently by men than by women and, if male unemployment continues to rise at a greater rate than female unemployment (albeit that women's jobs tend to be part time and relatively poorly paid), there is no doubt that such views will become increasingly pervasive. It is also likely that what has been termed the backlash to feminism will continue to receive media attention (Faludi, 1992).

Opposed to essentialist views are those accounts of gender which stress socialization and enculturation. From this perspective, many educationalists and social scientists will continue to point out the manner in which societies create differing destinies for males and females (Hargreaves and Colley, 1986). Feminists and social scientists coming from more structuralist perspectives (for example the social constructionist approach) will also continue to stress the manner in which 'masculine' behaviours and values continue to be overvalued (Hare-Mustin and Maracek, 1990).

This lack of academic and public consensus about issues of gender and gender identity has important implications for practitioners in the social and medical fields who must always be prepared to respond sensitively to the views of others even when such views radically transgress their own personal understandings of gender issues.

## Applications

### 1. Be non-judgemental
Gender identity and sexuality are intensely personal matters which few people are prepared to talk completely frankly about even to the most empathic of counsellors or health workers. Consequently those counselling clients need to be aware of their own attitudes to gender and sexuality and to indicate clearly that they are non-judgemental. Such a stance is more likely than any other to create trust and confidence.

### 2. Avoid making assumptions
Practitioners should also always ensure that they do not make assumptions about a client's sexuality.

### 3. Be sensitive to other cultures
Contemporary British society is multicultural, and culture conditions gender and gender identity. Practitioners working with clients from cultures with which they are relatively unfamiliar need to find out about notions of gender in those cultures and be sensitive to them.

### 4. Be aware of socioeconomic trends
Economic and social changes have dramatically affected relationships between the sexes and within families. Practitioners need to keep such trends firmly in view and avoid making assumptions about what is 'normal' within relationships or families.

# Further reading

Siann, G. (1994). *Gender, Sex and Sexuality: Contemporary Psychological Perspectives*. Brighton: Falmer.
Oskamp, S. and Costanzo, M. (eds) (1993). *Gender Issues in Contemporary Society*. Newbury Park, CA: Sage.

# References

Bandura, A. and Huston, A. C. (1961). Identification as a process of incidental learning. *Journal of Abnormal and Social Psychology*, **63**, 311–18.
Bandura, A. and Walters, R. H. (1963). *Social Learning and Personality Development*. New York: Holt, Rinehart and Winston.
Bem, S. (1983). Gender schema theory and its implications for child development: Raising gender-schematic children in a gender-schematic society. In *The Psychology of Women: Ongoing Debates* (M. R. Walsh, ed.) New Haven: Yale University Press.

Caplan, P. (ed.) (1987). *The Cultural Construction of Sexuality*. London: Tavistock.

Chodorow, N. (1979). Feminism and difference: Gender relation and difference in psychoanalytic perspective. *Socialist Review*, **46**, 42–64.

Deaux, K. (1987). Psychological constructions of masculinity and femininity. In *Masculinity/ Femininity: Basic Perspective* (J. M. Reinich and S. A. Saunders, eds) New York: Oxford University Press.

Ehrhardt, A. A. and Meyer-Bahlberg, H. F. L. (1981). Effects of prenatal sex hormones on gender related behavior. *Science*, **211**, 1312–18.

EOC (1992). *Women and Men in Britain 1992*, Equal Opportunities Commission.

Faludi, S. (1992). *Backlash: The Undeclared War against Women*. London: Vintage.

Fausto-Sterling, A. (1992). *Myths of Gender: Biological Theories about Men and Women*. 2nd edn, New York: Basic Books.

Foucault, M. (1979). *The History of Sexuality, Vol 1: An Introduction*. London: Allen Lane.

Fox, G. (1994). Till counselling us do part. *The Guardian*, 2, 21 Feb, pp. 6–7.

Garber, M. (1993). *Vested Interests: Cross Dressing and Cultural Anxiety*. Harmondsworth: Penguin.

Gilligan, C. (1982). *In a Different Voice*. Cambridge, Mass.: Cambridge University Press.

Hare-Mustin, R. T. and Maracek, J. (1990). *Making a Difference: Psychology and the Construction of Gender*. New Haven: Yale University Press.

Hargreaves, D. and Colley, A. M. (1986). *The Psychology of Sex Roles*. London: Harper and Row.

Hollway, W. (1989) *Subjectivity and Method in Psychology: Gender, Meaning and Science*. London: Sage.

James, L. and King, C. (1992). *Imagining Women: Cultural Representations and Gender*. Cambridge: Polity.

Kitzinger, C. (1992). Sandra Lipsitz Bem: feminist psychologist, *The Psychologist*, May, 222–4.

Kohlberg, L. (1966). A cognitive-developmental analysis of children's sex-role concepts and attitudes. In *The Development of Sex-Differences*. (E. E. Maccoby, ed.) Stanford: Stanford University Press.

Le Vay, S. (1993). *The Sexual Brain*. London: MIT Press.

Lyndon, N. (1992). *No More Sex Wars*. London: Sinclair-Stevenson.

Maccoby, E. E. and Jacklin, C. (1974). *The Psychology of Sex Differences*. Stanford: Stanford University Press.

MacDonald, M. (1995). *Representing Women: Myths of Feminity in the Popular Media*. London: Hodder & Stoughton.

Mitchell, J. (1974). *Psychoanalysis and Feminism*. Harmondsworth: Penguin.

Moore, S. (1994). No longer a man's man's man's world. *The Guardian*, 2, 18 Feb, p. 5.

Morris, J. (1974). *Conundrum*. New York: Harcourt, Brace, Jovanovich.

Parlee, M. B. (1985). Psychology of women in the 80s. Promising problems. *International Journal of Women's Studies*, **8**, pp. 193–204.

Piaget, J. (1954). *The Construction of Reality in the Child*. New York, Basic Books.

Roberts, Y. (1992). *Mad about Women: Can there ever be Fair Play between the Sexes?* London: Virago.

Rohrbaugh, J. (1981) *Women: Psychology's Puzzle*. London: Sphere.

Rossi, A. (1987). On the psychology of mothering. In *The Psychology of Women: Ongoing Debates* (M. R. Walsh, ed.) New Haven: Norton.

Ruse, N. (1988). *Homosexuality: A Philosophical Enquiry*. Oxford: Blackwell.

Rushton, J. P. (1992). Cranial capacity, related to sex, rank, and race in a stratified random sample of 6,325 US military personnel. *Intelligence*, **16**, 401–33.

Sanday, P. R. and Goodenough, R. G. (eds) (1990). *Beyond the Second Sex: New Directions in the Anthropology of Gender*, Philadelphia: University of Pennsylvania Press.

Sayers, J. (1992). *Mothering Psychoanalysis*. Harmondsworth: Penguin.

Siann, G. (1985). *Accounting for Aggression*. London: Allen and Unwin.

Siann, G. (1994). *Gender, Sex and Sexuality: Contemporary Psychological Perspectives*. Brighton: Falmer.

Siann, G. and Ugwuegbu, D. (1988). *Educational Psychology in a Changing World*. 2nd edn, London: Unwin Hyman.

Spence, J. T., Helmreich, R. L. and Stapp, J. (1975). Rating of self and peers on sex-role attributes and their relation to self-esteem and conceptions of masculinity and femininity. *Journal of Personality and Social Psychology*, **32**, 29–39.

Stanton, M. (1983). *Outside the Dream: Lacan and French Styles of Psychoanalysis*. London: Routledge and Kegan Paul.

Tavris, C. and Wade, C. (1984). *The Longest War: Sex Differences in Perspective*. 2nd edn, San Diego: Harcourt, Brace, Jovanovich.

Thomas, D. (1993). *Not Guilty: Men: The Case for the Defence*. London: Weidenfeld and Nicolson.

Tong, R. (1989). *Feminist Thought: A Comprehensive Introduction*. London: Routledge.

Unger, R. and Crawford, M. (1992). *Women and Gender: A Feminist Psychology*. London: McGraw-Hill.

Ussher, J. (1989). *The Psychology of the Human Body*. London: Routledge.

Williams, J. H. (1987). *The Psychology of Women: Behavior in a Biosocial Context*. 3rd edn, London: Norton.

Wilson, E. O. (1975). *Sociobiology: The New Synthesis*. Cambridge, Mass.: Harvard University Press.

Witkin, H. A., Mednick, S. A., Schulsinger, F. *et al.* (1976) Criminality in XYY and XXY men. *Science*, **193**, 547–55.

# 2

# Puberty and the psychosocial changes of adolescence

## Leo B. Hendry

Biological sex and psychosocial gender provide the backdrop for human reproduction. It is not until puberty, however, that both the physiological capacity to reproduce and the psychosocial awareness of reproductive potential emerge. Popular culture would have us believe that adolescence is a difficult time, full of conflict and intense emotion, and fraught with the potential for personal and societal harm – a time of 'storm and stress' – the awakening of sexuality and reproductive potential unleashing powerful forces which the adolescent may not have the psychological maturity to control. In this chapter, Leo Hendry asks whether adolescence is necessarily problematic and places puberty within its psychosocial context. Are adolescents at the mercy of their 'raging hormones' – or is reproductive capacity a more subtle influence on physiological and psychosocial development?

## Introduction

Stanley Hall's view of adolescence as a time of 'storm and stress' still maintains some currency in the general public's mind; as do Freud's ideas that adolescents' behaviour is motivated by unconscious psychosexual forces (Lloyd, 1985). More recently Davis (1990) has shown, by tracing historically the general public 'images' of adolescents in society, that themes of rebellion, moodiness and 'angst', delinquency, 'sinfulness', energy and excitement have been retained in adults' consciousness. Reinforced by images in the mass media this has created stereotyped pictures of youth in Britain today. There are current media fears about 'out-of-control' adolescents, joy-riders, delinquents, teenage mothers, 'lager-louts', drug abusers, punks and so on.

The social conventions of recent years have given adolescents greater self-determination at steadily younger ages and current social expectations for youth are remarkably problematic. This greater freedom for adolescents does carry with it more risks and costs of errors of judgement: 'dropping out' of school, being out of work, teenage pregnancy, sexually transmitted diseases, being homeless, drug addiction and suicide are powerful examples of the price that some young people pay for their extended freedom. The impact of making 'wrong' choices on individuals, families and wider society underscores the need for a better understanding of normal adolescent development and the transition to adulthood. Psychosocial theories of this transition emphasize the variety of 'tasks' that face adolescents in the process of growing up. Hence, the number and type of these adjustments and challenges have often been perceived to be at the root of the so-called 'storm and stress' of the teenage years. Given the rather negative public image of young people today, this chapter sets out to look at two key questions. Firstly, are puberty and adolescence problematic in present-day society? Secondly, what should be of concern to us about pubertal and psychosocial development in the adolescent's transition towards adulthood?

# Defining puberty and adolescence

## Physical and physiological changes of puberty

As Coleman and Hendry (1990) have outlined, some of the most important events to which young people have to adjust in the transition to adulthood are the multitude of physiological and morphological changes which are associated with puberty. The word puberty derives from the Latin 'pubertas', meaning age of manhood, and is usually considered to refer to the onset of menstruation in young women, and the emergence of pubic hair in young men (Coleman and Hendry, 1990). These two easily observable changes are only a small part of a complex process involving many bodily functions, which makes puberty itself difficult to define. Puberty is accompanied by changes not only in the reproductive system and in the secondary sexual characteristics of the individual, but in the size, weight and functioning of the heart and the accelerated growth of the lungs and thus of the cardiovascular system, in the size and the strength of many of the muscles of the body, a decline in basal metabolism, and so on. Puberty, therefore, can be seen as a physical event with wide-ranging psychosocial implications.

One of the many physical changes associated with puberty is the 'growth spurt'. This term is usually taken to refer to the accelerated rate of increase in height and weight that occurs during early adolescence. There are considerable individual differences in the age of onset and duration of the growth spurt among young people. In boys, the growth spurt may begin as early as 10 years of age, or as late as 16, while in girls the same process can begin at 7 or 8, or not until 12, 13 or even 14. For the average male, rapid growth begins at about 13, and reaches a peak somewhere during the fourteenth year. Comparable average ages for young women are 11 for the onset of the growth spurt, and 12 for the age of peak increase in height and weight (Tanner, 1978; Eveleth and Tanner, 1977). Noticeable to adolescents themselves, especially to young men, is an associated increase in physical strength and endurance (Coleman and Hendry, 1990).

Puberty also gives rise to less obvious internal changes which differ between men and women (e.g. Katchadourian, 1977). The pituitary gland is the regulator of the major physiological changes of early adolescence. This gland, located immediately below the brain, releases activating hormones. These in turn have a stimulating effect on most of the other endocrine glands, which then release their own growth-related hormones. Among the most important of these are the sex hormones, including testosterone in males and oestrogen in females, which stimulate the growth of mature sperm and ova. However, these hormones also combine with others such as thyroxine from the thyroid gland, and cortisol from the adrenal gland, to activate the growth of bone and muscle which leads to the growth spurt.

Changes in sexual characteristics are stimulated by activating hormones and occur, as with the growth spurt, approximately eighteen to twenty-four months later for young men than for young women. For males, the first sign of the approach of puberty is most commonly an increase in the rate of growth of the testes and scrotum, followed by the growth of the pubic hair. Acceleration of growth of the penis and the appearance of facial hair frequently accompany the beginning of the growth spurt. It is usually somewhat later than this that the voice breaks, and the first seminal discharge occurs. In females, enlargement of the breasts and the growth of pubic hair are early signs of puberty, and are followed by the development of the uterus and vagina. Menarche, the first menstruation, occurs relatively late in the developmental sequence, and almost always after the peak velocity of the growth spurt (Katchadourian, 1977).

The practical effects of this are that in young women the first event of puberty is often an increase in height which frequently passes unnoticed. In young men, on the other hand, peak height velocity usually occurs late in the sequence, and after pubic hair has appeared and genitalia have started to grow.

A variety of methods can be used to assess pubertal maturity. Measures of physical maturity are often needed by professionals who provide care to children and youths, and by those performing research involving adolescents. In pediatric situations stages of maturity can be assigned to secondary sex characteristics using the criteria popularized by Tanner (1962). Physical maturity can also be measured, through much longer age ranges, from standardized radiographs of particular bones or teeth (Roche, Wainer and Thissen, 1975; Demirjian, 1980). Other obvious indices of maturity level in young women relate to menarche. Serial data can be analysed in relation to intervals before and after menarche but only if age at menarche is known from inquiry close to the age of the event (Livson and McNeill, 1962). In many psychological studies, however, it may be impossible to assess pubertal stage by physical examination. Thus self-ratings and self-report scales combining a number of pubertal indices (Petersen, Crockett, Richards and Boxer, 1988) or pictures of the five pubertal stages described by Marshall and Tanner (1969, 1970) may be the only method of determining pubertal status. These use ratings of pubertal stage made by adolescents themselves or their parents (Brooks-Gunn, Warren, Rosso and Gargiuld, 1987). Such measures are generally non-invasive and may serve as reasonably valid and reliable indices of pubertal development (Petersen, 1988).

## Adolescence

Adolescence is as difficult to define as puberty. Within the teenage years, the adolescent becomes physically and sexually mature without necessarily being seen fully to assume adult social roles. Adolescence, as a time set aside for waiting, developing and maturing and for accomplishing the rites of passage between childhood and adult status, is an extended phase of life for today's young people. In the first place, no one is entirely sure when adolescence begins. For some it may be at 13, the first 'teen' year, while for others it may be at the start of secondary school. For those who prefer a physical marker the commencement of puberty is the obvious moment, yet puberty itself is a very complex phenomenon, with different elements – the growth spurt, menarche, and so on – occurring at different times. The picture is further confused by the so-called 'secular trend' in puberty, i.e. its occurrence approximately one month earlier in each decade of the twentieth century in western industrialized countries (Coleman and Hendry, 1990). Today a proportion of girls in the top classes of any primary school will have started puberty – are these 9, 10 or 11 year olds adolescent? Maturing to puberty at an earlier age than their parents and grandparents, young people become participants in domestic and global affairs through more open households and the omnipresent media. Thus today's child in some senses at least has entered upon adolescence long before leaving primary school. At the same time, however, compulsory schooling has been extended and the pressures on the workforce to become more skilled have put a premium on 'staying-on' at school or moving into tertiary education. The delay in acquiring an income is just one of the factors which seems to defer the passage to adulthood. The erosion of the traditional roles of the family, the church and the school – institutions originally associated with socialization of the young – has resulted in the fragmentation of the adolescent transition since various social environments function as independent, sometimes isolated and at times competitive or even contradictory settings for teenagers. It is this confusion of purpose at the community level and the disaffection which young people may develop towards it, rather than any nationwide rebelliousness towards adult society which create the possible conflicts of the adolescent identity crisis so frequently cited in the media (Coleman and Hendry, 1990). As Coleman (1979) has pointed out in emphasizing this period of the life cycle as socially contrived:

> Adolescence is a complex and contradictory stage of development. Adolescent behaviour itself is frequently paradoxical. For example, conformity may go hand-in-hand with rebellion, while spontaneity alternates with sullen reserve....A spirit of fierce independence is transformed in the space of a few minutes into childish dependence, yet the most difficult teenager may become, almost overnight, a delightful and rewarding companion. Equally confusing are the discrepancies which exist between the images of young people as they are presented in newspapers, or on film and television, and the behaviour of the great majority of adolescents in our society. On the one hand it must seem from the media as if there is no escape from the anger, violence and mindless drifting of the younger generation, yet on the other hand countless hard-working or exam-orientated teenagers are in evidence in every neighbourhood.

## Experiencing puberty

The physiological changes discussed above inevitably exercise a profound effect upon the individual. The body alters radically in size and shape, and it is not surprising that many adolescents experience a period of clumsiness as they attempt to adapt to these changes. The body also alters in function, and new and sometimes worrying physical experiences such as the girl's first period, or the boy's nocturnal emissions, have to be understood. Perhaps most important of all, however, is the effect that such physical changes have upon identity. As many writers have pointed out, the development of the individual's identity requires not only the notion of being separate and different from others, but also a sense of self-consistency, and a firm knowledge of how one appears to the rest of the world (e.g. Rosenberg, 1979). Dramatic bodily changes seriously affect those aspects of identity and represent a considerable challenge in adaptation for even the most well-adjusted young person.

Experimental evidence has clearly shown that the average adolescent is not only sensitive to, but often critical of, his or her changing physical self (Davies and Furnham, 1986). Thus, probably largely as a result of the importance of films and television, teenagers tend to have idealized norms for physical attractiveness, and to feel inadequate if they do not match these unrealistic criteria. Lerner and Karabenick (1974) showed that adolescents who perceived themselves to deviate physically from cultural stereotypes were likely to have impaired self-concepts, and many other studies have pointed out the important role that physical characteristics play in determining self-esteem, especially in the younger adolescent (Rosenberg, 1979). Simmons and Rosenberg (1975) have reported studies in which North American adolescents were asked what they did and did not like about themselves. Results showed that those in early adolescence used primarily physical characteristics to describe themselves, and it was these characteristics which were most often disliked. It was not until later adolescence that intellectual or social aspects of personality were widely used in self description, but these characteristics were much more frequently liked than disliked. It is therefore just at the time of most rapid physical change that appearance is of critical importance for the individual, both for his or her self-esteem as well as for popularity. These findings were very similar to those reported by Hendry, Shucksmith, Love and Glendinning (1993) within a seven-year longitudinal study of British adolescents.

Since individuals mature at very different rates, one young woman at the age of 14 may be small, and look very much as she did during childhood, while another of the same age may look like a fully-developed adult woman. The question arises as to whether such marked physical differences have particular consequences for the individual's psychological adjustment. By and large longitudinal studies have shown that, for adolescent males, early maturation carries with it social advantages, while late maturation can be more of a problem. In comparison with early maturers, late maturing young men have been found to be less relaxed, less popular, more dependent and less attractive to both adults and peers (Mussen and Jones, 1957; Clausen, 1975). The picture for adolescent women, however, is more complex, for early maturation seems to have both costs and benefits. As a number of writers have shown, those who mature early are less popular with their peers, and more likely to show signs of inner turbulence than those who mature later (e.g. Peskin, 1973). On the other hand it has also been reported that early maturation can lead to enhanced self-confidence and social prestige (Clausen, 1975). Similarly Clausen (1975) indicated that social class was significant, with middle-class early maturers being at a greater advantage than their working-class peers.

Two particular topics addressed by Brooks-Gunn (1987) and Petersen (1988) were the meaning of puberty for the individual and those in his or her immediate social environment, and the factors which affect the timing of puberty. Of importance here is the deviance hypothesis within a lifespan developmental approach (Petersen and Crockett, 1985) which states that early and late maturers differ from on-time maturers because of their status, being socially deviant compared to their peer group. This hypothesis predicts that early maturing girls and late maturing boys are at risk for adjustment problems because they constitute the two most deviant groups in terms of maturation.

Stattin and Magnusson (1990) have commented on the effects of maturational timing on adolescent young women. Early maturers reported weight problems and expressed dissatisfaction with their temperament. They also reported more problems in relationships with their parents, especially with their mothers, and with adult authority figures such as teachers. Timing of maturation was also related to patterns of same-sex relationships, with early developers preferring to associate with other early developers, and late developers with late peers. Early maturing women associated with older young men, were exposed to sexual experience at a younger age than other young women and were more likely to have had an abortion during the teenage years.

Similarly, Silbereisen and Noack (1990) have found that early maturation is likely to be positive for young men, but negative for young women. In this study, early maturing adolescent young women were more likely to associate with older males, to be unpopular with female age mates and to use cigarettes and alcohol regularly. Similarly late maturers, both young men and young women, were likely to be at a disadvantage in comparison with 'on-time' adolescents in a wide range of areas of development. Rodriguez-Tomé and Bariaud (1990) have focused on three main areas of psychological development in relation to biological development during early adolescence, namely cognitive processes, self-concept and socio-emotional reactions. Their findings show that as maturation progresses young women evaluate their physical attractiveness but not their physical condition more negatively than young men. Young men's evaluation of their relationships with young women improves with physical maturation whereas adolescent women's evaluations of relationships with young men remain more or less constant throughout the maturational period.

## Identity

Pubertal changes attract the attention of the adolescent to his or her own body because they raise the issue of identity. Adolescents observe changes, evaluate them, attempt to integrate them in a personal 'style' and invite (sometimes even challenge) others, more or less consciously, to be involved in the quest for identity, since identity is not just 'for oneself', but also 'for others' (Goffman, 1971; Rodriguez-Tomé, 1972).

'Body image', therefore, is not a reflection of the body *as it is*, but interpretations of it. These interpretations are influenced by individual factors and by contextual ones such as meanings and values which the culture confers on masculine and feminine physiques (Lerner, 1985; Coleman and Hendry, 1990; Bruchon-Schweitzer, 1990).

Adolescents, because of sexual and gender development, are inevitably confronted, perhaps for the first time, with cultural standards of beauty and attractiveness in relation to evaluating 'body image'. The influence of these standards may come to the individual directly, for instance via media images or by the reactions of others (e.g. Eagly, Ashmore, Makhijani and Longo, 1991). Research on 'body image' suggests that, in contrast to men, adolescent and adult women frequently express dissatisfaction with their body shape and weight (Fallon and Rozin, 1985, in the USA; Tiggemann and Pennington, 1990, in Australia). Many North American young women judged that they were too fat, even when they were in fact of average build or thin. This was particularly true if they came from middle class or wealthy upper class backgrounds (Duncan, Ritter, Dornbusch et al., 1985). Adolescent (and adult) men in this study did not have the same desire – and were not subject to the same social pressures – to be slim, unless they were particularly overweight, though many of them would have liked to be more muscular (Duncan, Ritter, Dornbusch et al., 1985). The concern of young women with their weight is frequently accompanied by dieting practices, and sometimes by serious eating disorders (Greenfeld, Quinlan, Harding et al., 1987; Ledoux, Choquet and Flament, 1991).

The impact of puberty on body images varies with gender (Crockett and Petersen, 1987; Nottelmann, Susman, Inoff-Germain et al., 1987). Dissatisfaction with weight seems to be an effect of maturation *per se*, because it goes with an increase in adipose tissue in women, whereas in males it is associated with an increase in muscularity (Duncan, Ritter, Dornbusch et al., 1985). In late adolescence, early developers are also less satisfied with their body shape (Simmons, Blyth and McKinney, 1983). Similarly, Tobin-Richards, Boxer and Petersen (1983) found that young women who were 'on-time' had the most positive feelings about their bodies, late developers viewed themselves less positively, whilst early developers had the most negative self-perceptions.

## Menarche

Ruble and Brooks-Gunn (1982) have claimed that adolescent women's reactions to menarche reflect mixed emotional reactions. Whilst they are concerned to keep the fact of menstruation secret, especially from their fathers and other males, they are also proud of 'becoming a woman'. The overall pattern of results in this study suggests that initially menarche may create inconvenience, ambivalence and confusion, especially for early-maturing and unprepared girls, but that it is not as traumatic as may be held in popular belief. However, a study by Stoltzman (1986) found that adolescents were more likely to view menstruation as debilitating, bothersome and unsanitary and less likely to view it as a positive event than their mothers. Adolescents reported significantly more acute pain, water retention and arousal symptoms around menstruation than did their mothers.

From a psychodynamic perspective, Teja (1976) considered that menarche, as a manifest event, makes it imperative for the developing adolescent girl to face her sexuality and deal with it. He argued that sexual drives are heightened at this time, and that the ego must handle them through adaptive processes of either partial or complete gratification or sublimation.

Menstrual bleeding can have a variety of cultural and symbolic meanings, one of which is its perception as a 'curse' (Delaney, Lupton and Toth, 1988). Several factors can reduce the effect of such negative stereotypes on the experience of menarche, and some can even make it more positive. These include preparation for both the physical and psychological aspects of the event, and learning to believe that changes are a normal part of development. Timing is also important; knowing that one 'fits in' with others can be comforting to adolescents. Factors influencing the psychological impact of menarche include age at time of first period, social factors, amount of preparation, and cultural factors including lay beliefs (Clarke and Ruble, 1978).

## Experiencing adolescence

The variety of psychosocial 'tasks' to be achieved in the adolescent transition – personal development, social relationships, leaving school, seeking qualifications and employment (or finding unemployment), leisure pursuits, creating a particular lifestyle, becoming mature and independent – are all relevant to reproductive psychology and important to understand. In this section of the present chapter only two aspects, namely relationships and sexuality and gender, are discussed to illustrate certain key elements which may be of relevance to the various facets of the total transition from puberty to adulthood.

# Relationships

Coleman and Hendry (1990) have proposed that at different times during adolescence particular sorts of relationship patterns come into focus. They suggest that concern about gender role peaks around 13 years; concerns about acceptance by or rejection from peers are highly important around 15 years; while issues regarding the gaining of independence from parents climb steadily to peak beyond 16 years and then begin to tail off. It seems clear, for example, that the influence of peers peaks in mid-adolescence, and this suggests that young people would be particularly susceptible at this stage to peer group pressures of various kinds. This is supported to some extent by a seven-year longitudinal study of lifestyle development (Hendry, Shucksmith, Love and Glendinning, 1993) which showed that independence of thought and action began to emerge from mid to late adolescence as concerns regarding peer acceptance lessen.

Clearly entry into a new phase in the life course challenges self-identity and particularly individual self-evaluations as young people attempt new tasks in which they can succeed or fail; as they alter their values and the areas which are important for overall self-esteem; and as they confront new significant others against whom they rate themselves and about whose judgements they care. Rosenberg (1979) has emphasized the importance of the reflected self and of social comparison in determining self-esteem as well as the importance of doing well in the areas one values (i.e. his principle of psychological centrality).

During adolescence clear changes take place in relationship patterns. Greater significance is given to peers as companions, as providers of advice, support and feedback, as models for behaviour and as sources of comparative information concerning personal qualities and skills. Relationships with parents alter in the direction of greater equality and reciprocity (Coleman and Hendry, 1990; Hendry, Shucksmith, Love and Glendinning, 1993) and parental authority comes to be seen as an area which is itself open to discussion and negotiation (Youniss and Smollar, 1990) and within which discriminations can be made (Coleman and Coleman, 1984). Fend (1990) investigated the relationship between ego strength development and social relationships, and showed that a decline in ego strength over time is related to a growing social gap between parents and peers. He also showed that the parent/adolescent relationship is more important than peer relationships for ego strength development. However, both types of relationships are of importance for coping successfully with the developmental tasks of adolescents in that both contribute to a positive self-concept. The significance of both types of relationships is supported by research carried out by Palmonari, Pombeni and Kirchler (1989). Part of this work involved examining how Italian adolescents used different relationships in order to deal with various types of problem they encounter. A traditional (storm and stress) model would predict a straightforward change from 'reference to parents' to 'reference to peers' as adolescence progresses. In fact, the study showed that young people act in a selective way; depending on the type of problem reference could be made to parents, to peers or to both. Similar findings have been demonstrated in a Dutch study by Meeus (1989) and in a Scottish study by Hendry, Shucksmith, Love and Glendinning (1993).

Family itself is increasingly being recognized as a more complex and variable entity than the statistical caricature of two parents and two point four children. In

Britain at least 20 per cent of children, and in the USA a much higher figure, will grow up in 're-constituted' families. The varieties of family forms, patterns, and styles of relationships all have their strengths and weaknesses, and some 'fit' better with some young people, while others fit better with others.

Hendry (1993) has suggested that the changing social scene has, in some senses, 'de-skilled parents' simply because they no longer have direct experience themselves of some of the social contexts and behaviours that their adolescent children are experiencing and therefore feel unable to, and lack confidence in, giving advice to their family beyond general views regarding the legality of particular behaviours and about personal moral values. With regard to parenting styles and their influence, Hendry, Shucksmith, Love and Glendinning (1993) have shown their importance to adolescent physical and mental health and to the development of lifestyle. One particular parenting style seemed to have important effects even after a number of years, including an influence on mental health. The neglectful family stood out as quite distinct from other types. Adolescents growing up within this parenting style were more likely to spend more time with their peer group than other adolescents and they had very negative attitudes to school as well as to the family itself. They were also more likely to feel peer pressure to drink and smoke and to regard theft and vandalism as justified within certain circumstances. Although they spent long periods with friends they did not regard themselves as easy to get along with and they were more likely to report psychological stress.

Parents can be uneasy in discussing developmental concerns with their teenage offspring. In a longitudinal study (Hendry, Shucksmith, Love and Glendinning, 1993), the most startling differences between boys and girls were in the realm of discussions about the more intimate matters, such as problems with friends, self-doubt, views about sex and so on. Nearly 70 per cent of all girls chose to confide in their mother over problems with friends, and 41.2 per cent of the boys preferred to speak to their mother about such matters. Fathers were the choice of only 3.9 per cent of the girls and 11.1 per cent of the boys in this matter. Doubts about their own abilities would be voiced to their mother by nearly half the girls and 33.2 per cent of the boys. Only 16.1 per cent of girls and 26.5 per cent of boys would speak to their fathers about a similar concern. Figures like these point to a disengagement by these fathers from the affairs of most concern to their adolescent children in these years of critical development.

Girls tend to be very uncomfortable talking to their fathers about pubertal issues across adolescence and learn almost nothing about puberty from their fathers (less than 15 per cent tell their fathers when they reach menarche; Brooks-Gunn, 1987). These findings suggest that father–daughter discussions regarding a daughter's pubertal developments are rare. Family openness about daughter's menarche, even if it provokes anger or bickering in early adolescence, may have more long-term positive values. In a study of eleventh- and twelfth-grade girls, those who reported that their fathers knew about their menarche early (generally from the mother) had less negative attitudes about their bodies and menstruation than those who reported their fathers did not hear about their menarche (Brooks-Gunn, 1987). Ease in discussing sexual issues with the mother has also been associated with more consistent contraceptive use in older adolescents (Fox, 1981).

## Peers, gender and sexuality

The peer group provides the adolescent with comparison references, sends back images of himself or herself and enables him or her to experience new forms of friendship and intimacy (Coleman and Hendry, 1990). Roles become increasingly sex typed with the sexual maturation of the body which occurs at puberty and sexual differences become more significant and pervasive in social situations. The period of separation of the sexes around the late primary school stage and the start of adolescence is followed by an interest in peers of the opposite sex and the desire for closeness with them. Establishment of relations with the opposite sex is another major developmental task of adolescence (Havighurst, 1972).

A few studies have investigated the influence of pubertal development on relations with peers of the same sex and the opposite sex. Different aspects of these relations have been studied in terms of behaviour and perceptions. Findings indicate that girls who develop earlier are more involved than others in heterosexual relationships, during early or mid-adolescence (Magnusson, Stattin and Allen, 1985, in Sweden; Simmons and Blyth, 1987, in the USA). As to perceptions of relationships, the work of Simmons, Blyth and McKinney (1983) on American girls suggests that physical maturation leads to an increase in girls' feeling that they are popular in the eyes of boys, and in the importance which they attribute to this.

A study by Streitmatter (1985) found that male and female gender identification prior to adolescence was fairly distinct. Entry into adolescence seemed to cloud the issue. The pattern indicated decreasing differentiation from 12 to 13, 13 to 14, and 14 to 15 years. However, 15 to 16 year old comparisons reflected increasing differentiation. Apparently, gender identifications which are adopted in childhood are reconsidered and reformulated during adolescence. Gilligan (1990) contended that as girls enter adolescence they seriously confront the disadvantages of their gender and suffer from a lack of confidence and a confused sense of identity. A second watershed appears to be the transition from school to work when girls discover how limited their occupational prospects are in contrast to boys and they begin to have to make hard choices about career and personal life that belie the notion of an easy combination of work and family (see Chapter 1).

By puberty, most children will have a relatively secure view of themselves as male or female, as defined in the particular culture in which the child develops. In adolescence, the task of resolving the issues of identity includes that of sexual identity. Masculinity and femininity have to be renegotiated in adolescent terms, a significant portion of which concern sexuality, which previously had little relevance to gender (Bancroft, 1990). The child enters adolescence with the elements necessary for sexual orientation, rather than sexual orientation *per se*. Thus sexual identity is intimately connected to how gender identity is perceived within the culture. Goldman and Goldman (1982) argue that physiology creates only the potential for sexual behaviour; actual behaviour is principally organized by social roles. This view is supported by Hampson and Money's (1955) study of the sexual thinking of children with hormonal anomalies. These children, having a precocious puberty, thought about sex in a way that was congruent with their peers rather than in tune with the level of their physiological development.

As Bancroft (1990) has stressed, sexual behaviour and experimentation in adolescence is the medium through which gender identity is reorganized, rather than being a simple function of physiological development. It is when the development of identity (both gender and otherwise) is out of step (for whatever reason) with the development of sexual ideation and fantasy that a young person is likely to be disturbed by the experience. Sexual exploration does not need to conform to any particular prescribed age or phase. Although it includes physical and sexual experimentation in its own right, the predominant feature is the experimentation with new experiences in the context of a new identity. Thus experimentation is partly being in the role of a sexual person, both in the eyes of him/herself, of potential partners, and of peers and rivals, and partly exploring new kinds of relationships and the possibility of feeling often previously taboo emotions in the context of those relationships. It is not therefore surprising that young people may try a number of different sexual roles, the nature of which will be closely connected to their attempts to develop some separate identity in the context of, and sometimes in opposition to, their families. Experimentation often includes, at least in fantasy, experimenting with gender roles. From a developmental point of view sexual variations, including homosexuality, or attraction to older men or women, are not necessarily a reason for concern. They are best considered in terms of the young person exploring which 'elements' of sexual orientation are to become his or hers.

The adolescent sexual experience in the 1990s is unlike the experience of any adult – parent or grandparent. It is now accompanied by the threat of the human immunodeficiency virus (HIV) (see Chapter 10). Thus, given that adolescence starts five years earlier and that marriage takes place six or seven years later than it did 100 years ago, our public policy on sex education, contraception, and abortion is regrettably blind to the realities of sexuality for individuals within this eleven-year extended adolescence.

Bakken and Romig (1992) have suggested that educational programmes should emphasize and provide for the development of understanding intimacy and leadership in adolescent relationships because there is a need to enable young males in particular to develop relationship styles based less on hierarchy and more on interaction and intimacy. In terms of addressing leadership within relationships, programmes that encourage assertiveness would be helpful to young women. Such programmes could also benefit adolescents by helping them to learn to balance leadership and intimacy needs in relationships so that neither is sacrificed to gain the other. It is clear from our own studies on young people and sexual relationships (Hendry, Shucksmith, Philip and Jones, 1991) that power and intimacy are two dimensions around which young people need guidance and help to understand the ways in which romantic and sexual relationships are negotiated.

In present day society a tremendous strain may be put on some adolescents in developing sexual relationships. Sexual role identity is very important during adolescence, yet societal changes do not occur evenly, so adolescents may be caught in possible paradoxes of male/female differences and chastity/sexuality dilemmas. Cultural influences can be a powerful determinant of these paradoxes. Society places great value on adolescents' physical development and in turn they judge themselves in relation to these responses, feeling rejected or of low value if they do not conform to social ideals.

In certain settings peer pressure may create a conflict between what the individual adolescent believes and what many of his or her friends are doing. Because peers play such an important role in the lives of adolescents, social acceptance and social relations are likely to be urgent concerns for most young people. In Hendry, Shucksmith, Philip and Jones' (1991), study young women were found to adopt a number of techniques for avoiding potentially difficult situations: for some, limiting their alcohol intake was an important mechanism although this in itself could pose problems of being seen as lacking in fun, and becoming a figure of ridicule. Pubs were viewed by the majority of young people as essential features of social life whether alcohol was used or not, but leaving the pub was where difficulties arose for many young women. Some avoided parties in houses unless they went with a boyfriend who could afford them some protection. Others who were of age to drive would see the use of a car as an acceptable means of avoidance which would not jeopardize membership of a particular peer group. For many young women, fear of loss of sexual reputation was uppermost in their minds in relation to risk-taking behaviour. In this context alcohol and drug taking were viewed as disinhibitors and likely to lead to loss of control of situations, and the consequences could be serious. However, to avoid alcohol use in particular was liable to lead to exclusion from social activities and isolation so a balance had to be struck. In relation to safer sex, carrying condoms was perceived as inappropriate and likely to suggest a girl was 'looking for it', leaving her open to abuse. As one young woman said in the study: 'You'll get AIDS and cancer if you use the pill and slagged off if you carry a condom!'

One group of girls complained that boys routinely went through their bags at discos and would perceive the existence of condoms to imply the girl was promiscuous. Among this group of girls such intrusion was an accepted aspect of their lives which they faced not with contempt but resignation.

Young men also have developmental concerns which stem from puberty. Rites of passage into manhood are under pressure in this time of rapid social change, with mass youth unemployment, radically changing family forms, increased consumer pressures and an influential popular culture that informs young people's emotional and sexual lives. These are the processes within which gender apprenticeships are played out in homes, peer groups and workplaces. Males are not passively socialized into fixed gender and sexual roles. Rather they are actively engaged in making gender identities, in which they have deep cultural investments. Of particular significance is the danger of the learning of a masculine code, which separates sexual practices from emotional feelings. Hence we need to recognize more clearly how economic and social changes can affect young men's gender development and responsibilities in relation to future domestic roles.

## Theoretical explanations of adolescent experiences

From the pubertal changes that herald the teenage years, the adolescent has various personal and social 'learning' tasks to achieve. Havighurst (1972) proposed a range of such psychosocial tasks in adolescence and early adulthood (Table 2.1). There are, however, no symbolic 'rites of passage' in western society, so the adolescent's route towards adulthood is not marked out by clearly defined signposts which indicate progress in a desired direction. A

**Table 2.1** The personal and social learning tasks of adolescence

| Adolescence (12–18 years) | | Early adulthood (18–30 years) | |
|---|---|---|---|
| 1 | Achieving new and more mature relations with the age mates of both sexes | 1 | Selecting a mate |
| 2 | Achieving a masculine or feminine social role | 2 | Learning to live with a marriage partner |
| 3 | Accepting one's physique and using the body effectively | 3 | Starting a family |
| 4 | Achieving emotional independence of parents | 4 | Rearing children |
| 5 | Preparing for marriage and family life | 5 | Managing a home |
| 6 | Preparing for an economic career | 6 | Getting started in an occupation |
| 7 | Acquiring a set of values and an ethical system as a guide to behaviour – developing an ideology | 7 | Taking on civic responsibility |
| 8 | Desiring and achieving socially responsible behaviour | 8 | Finding a congenial social group |

*Source*: Based on Havighurst (1972)

number of fairly recent theoretical explanations and major metatheories have been advanced to underpin our understanding of the adolescent transition from puberty to adulthood, and these are briefly described below.

### Psychoanalytic approach

The psychoanalytic approach deals with the individual in terms of maturation, physical and psychological development, and individuation, a process which 'involves the growing person in taking increasing responsibility for what he/she is and for what he/she does' (Blos, 1967). Individuation, however, necessarily involves disengagement from earlier childhood attachments. Blos (1962) has described adolescence as a 'second individuation process', the first having been completed towards the end of the third year of life. In his view both periods have certain things in common: there is an urgent need for psychological changes which help the individual adapt to maturation; there is an increased vulnerability of personality; and finally, both periods are followed by specific psychopathology should the individual run into difficulties.

The process of individuation is dependent upon the severance of childhood emotional attachments; however, these attachments can only be surrendered, so it is believed, by a reanimation of infantile involvements and patterns of behaviour. As Blos (1967) explains: 'The adolescent has to come into emotional contact with the passions of his infancy and early childhood in order for them to surrender their original cathexes; only then can the past fade into conscious and unconscious memories.'

One final matter associated with disengagement needs to be mentioned as an integral feature of the psychoanalytic view of adolescence. Blos (1967) believes that the adolescent need for intense emotional states, including delinquent activities, drug and mystical experiences, and short-lived but intense relationships, may be seen as a means of coping with inner emptiness. Blos includes here the need to do things 'just for kicks', which he argues simply represents a way of combating the emotional flatness, depression, and loneliness which are part of the separation experience.

Thus the psychoanalytic approach concentrates on the psychosexual factors and internal forces which underlie the young person's movement away from childhood behaviour and emotional involvement (see Chapter 1).

## Lifespan approach

A lifespan approach to human development stresses the dynamic interaction in the socialization process and draws attention to the adolescent in three modes: as stimulus (eliciting different reactions from the social environment); as processor, in making sense of the behaviour of others; and as agent, shaper and selector, by doing things, making choices and influencing events. These ideas concerning reciprocal influences and individual young people as 'active agents' in their own transitional process from childhood to adulthood (Lerner, 1985) are important theoretical themes in gaining an understanding of young people.

Erikson (1968) suggested that there are eight psychosocial crises extending through the individual's lifespan which establish stages in the development of personal maturity. He also suggested that the search for identity becomes especially acute during adolescence as a result of rapid changes in the biological, social and psychological aspects of the individual, and because of the necessity for occupational decisions to be made, ideals to be accepted or rejected and sexual and friendship choices to be determined. Erikson's view was that, as far as adolescence is concerned, the chief task involves the establishment of a *coherent identity*, and the defeat of a sense of *identity diffusion*; while Laufer and Laufer (1985) believed that the development of sexual identity specifically is what makes adolescence a psychological experience quite separate from childhood and the adult years.

A period of psychosocial moratorium during which decisions are left in abeyance may occur. This may allow the young person to delay major identity choices and experiment with roles in order to discover the sort of person he or she wishes to be; while such a stage may lead to disorientation or disturbance it has, according to Erikson, a healthy function.

## Biological approach

The biological approach has mainly focused on puberty and attributes the psychological experiences of adolescence to changing hormone levels. From the young person's perspective, biology may significantly underpin their changing attitudes to parental authority. Firstly, increased concentration or fluctuation in hormonal levels may affect parent–adolescent relationships directly. Changes in hormone concentration or variability could heighten the adolescent's arousal or emotional ability so that his or her responses to parent initiatives are more negative or unexpected, resulting in less predictable and potentially more volatile parent–child interactions (Paikoff and Brooks-Gunn, 1990; Steinberg, 1987).

Secondly, the hormonal changes of puberty could affect adolescent and parent behaviour through the creation of the young person's secondary sex characteristics and the other physical changes of puberty. These changes are salient to both adolescent and parent, and they signal the reproductive and social maturity of the young person, an event laden with meaning for both (Brooks-Gunn and Zahaykevich, 1989; Collins, 1990).

## Sociological/social–psychological approach

Sociological and social–psychological approaches see the causes of the adolescent's transition towards adulthood to lie primarily in social contexts. They concentrate on socialization, role development and role conflict, the acquisition of new roles and adaptation to new skills, the pressures of social expectations, and on the relative influence of various socializing agents which hurry or delay this move towards maturity. From this perspective it may be thought that the development of role behaviour is largely determined by an interaction between the adolescent's relationships with 'significant others' and his or her perceptions of the expectations of those 'others'. It is thought that adolescents are exposed to agents of socialization – peers, education system, the mass media, and political institutions all pulling in different directions; or that increasing age segregation in society means there is less opportunity for some young people to be in contact with adult models, and so the transition to maturity and the assumption of adult roles is made problematic. This viewpoint would regard adolescence less as an internal developmental process, and more as a social construct (Coleman and Hendry, 1990).

Thus, the sociological or socio–psychological approach to adolescence is marked by a concern with roles and role change, and with the processes of socialization. There can be little doubt that adolescence, from this point of view, is seen as being dominated by stresses and tensions, not so much because of inner emotional instability, but as a result of conflicting pressures from outside.

## Focal, social and economic theories

A more integrated theory of development is required in order to reconcile these dramatically different views of adolescence. Because of the complexities of modern society, children can reach physical adulthood before many of them are capable of functioning well in adult social roles. The disjunction between physical capabilities and socially approved independence and power, and the concurrent status ambiguities, can be stressful for the self-image of the adolescent.

Coleman (1979) presented a 'focal theory' arguing that the transition between childhood and adulthood cannot be achieved without substantial adjustments of both a psychological and social nature. Nevertheless, despite the amount of overall change experienced, most young people are extremely resilient and appear to cope with adjustments without undue stress.

Coleman's 'focal theory' offers a reason or rationale for this apparent contradiction. In it he proposes that at different ages particular sorts of relationship patterns come into focus, in the sense of being most prominent, but that no pattern is specific to one age only. Thus the patterns overlap, different issues come into focus at different times, but simply because an issue is not the most prominent feature at a particular age does not mean that it may not be critical for some individuals. These ideas, derived from empirical findings, combine to suggest a symbolic model of adolescent development where each curve represents a different issue or relationship. This is illustrated in Figure 2.1.

This theory focusses on psychological–rational issues and concerns rather than on wider social factors. However, if an adolescent girl sees herself as an adult while her parents still see her as a child, or if an adolescent boy perceives

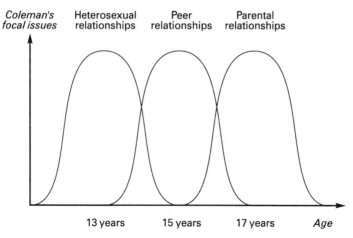

*Coleman's*    Heterosexual     Peer      Parental
*focal issues*   relationships   relationships  relationships

13 years     15 years     17 years    *Age*

**Figure 2.1** The 'focal theory' model. *Source*: Coleman (1979)

himself as weak and skinny while acceptance by the peer group requires aggressive masculinity, then there is conflict or dissonance (Hendry, 1983). This would suggest that external social factors are just as important as personal psychological ones in determining social, relational behaviour. Feedback, on which self-concept is dependent, may be positive or negative and will consequently result in consonance or dissonance. It is this dimension which Coleman's original focal model appears to omit. Feedback can lead to learning and subsequently to altered behaviour and to the development of a more stable self-concept via altered attitudes and beliefs (though of course in its turn feedback can be ignored and not acted upon!).

Other theories (Coffield, Borrill and Marshall, 1986 – Figure 2.2) have suggested that economic factors such as disadvantage and deprivation may have an all-pervading influence which determines to a large extent the options and choices available to young people in underprivileged sections of society. There can be little doubt that in situations of economic hardship it will be more difficult to manage the adolescent transitions in a satisfactory manner. This point has already been made by Hendry (1983) in his argument that ecological factors are as important as psychological ones in understanding the young person's development. However, focal theory has to do with the psychological transitions of adolescence rather than with the economic and social circumstances of the individual *per se*. For example, all young people, irrespective of social background, attempt to negotiate increasing independence from their parents. The focal model suggests that it will be easier to handle the parental issue if the young person is not, at the same time, striving for greater acceptance within the peer group. Teenagers are less able to cope if at one and the same time they are uncomfortable, for example with their bodies, owing to physical changes; with family, owing to changes in the family constellation; with home, because of a move; with school, owing to great discontinuity in the nature of the school environment; or with peers, because of disruption of peer networks and changes in peer expectations and peer evaluation criteria, and because of the emergence of opposite-sex relationships.

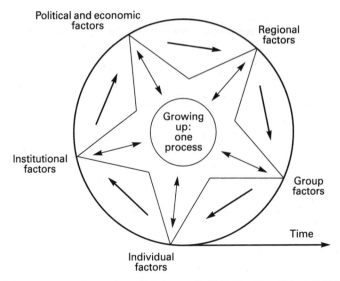

**Figure 2.2** An attempt at an integrating model. *Source*: Coffield, Burrill and Marshall (1986)

## Summary and conclusions

As we have seen in this chapter, puberty is the process by which children reach reproductive maturity, and it consists of a number of interdependent biological processes, ranging from the purely physiological (e.g. hormonal changes) to the physical (e.g. pubic hair growth and vaginal or testicular development) to the psychosocial (i.e. changes that are visible to others, such as breast growth or facial hair and which have social meaning). The onset of such a process links with the adolescent's transition from childhood towards adulthood and social maturity, and embodies the various psychosocial 'tasks' discussed in the chapter. Many of the studies reveiwed here confirm that adolescence does not inevitably spell trouble or difficulty for the majority of young people, though there is also evidence that adolescents' moods, self-consciousness and behaviour can differ from those of children and adults in certain ways.

The chapter concluded by offering a number of theoretical perspectives which can (hopefully) lead us towards a better understanding of the effects of puberty on adolescents' psychosocial development. As Offer and Offer (1975) suggested two decades ago, early adolescence may be a time of both adjustment and vulnerability.

There is evidence of psychological, social and behavioural adjustments having to be made during the early adolescent/pubertal years in the areas of self-consciousness and family relationships. Of course, many changes take place in early adolescence – including school transition and external bodily changes as well as increased concentrations of and fluctuation in hormones.

The importance of understanding biological underpinnings of pubertal development is vital to our knowledge of the onset of the adolescent years. The internal forces considered by a psychoanalytic approach, and sociological/ social–psychological interest in social roles and expectations, lets us examine 'both sides of the coin' so to speak, in understanding the adolescent's learning of appropriate social roles in various contexts whilst retaining individuality and 'selfhood'. These are the 'push–pull' mechanisms of inner drives and external social pressures within the adolescent transition.

According to person–environment 'fit' theory (Eccles and Midgley, 1989), behaviour, motivation, and mental health are influenced by the 'goodness of fit' between the characteristics individuals bring to their social environments and the characteristics of these social environments. Thus Coffield, Borrill and Marshall's (1986) model reminds us of the broader social and cultural factors which impact on the transition to adulthood in the various developmental domains; while Lerner (1985) stresses the dynamic interactions in the socialization process whereby the individual can be an 'active agent' in his/her own development and can be provided (to some extent) with a personal 'locus of control'. Young people do play an active role in choosing and shaping the contexts in which they operate and develop friendships, activities and lifestyles.

At the core of these interrelated – yet different – theories lies a central theme concerning the resolution of psychosocial issues across the adolescent years. Thus perhaps puberty and the adolescent transition can best be understood through a modified focal theory approach. Coleman and Hendry (1990) suggested that concern about gender roles and the initial learning about relationships with the opposite sex declines from a peak around 13 years; concerns about acceptance by or rejection from peers are highly important around 15 years; while issues regarding the gaining of independence from parents climb steadily to peak beyond 16 years. It is important to note the co-temporality of the onset of puberty with the first of these focal issues, namely concerns with seeking a gender identity and the commencement of adult-like relationships with peers and the opposite sex. This is the first phase of the intertwining of pubertal and adolescent development. From this largely observational phase (in social learning terms), the young person moves on to a 'rehearsal' stage of social skills, roles and strategies, mostly associated with peer acceptance and peer involvement before 'trying out' these behaviours and roles for their acceptance in adult society. The third focal 'step' sees the young person being more accepted into, and more comfortable in, various adult social contexts and settings such as clubs and pubs, entering the labour market, having longer-term 'responsible' relationships, and developing a maturity of outlook. From the starting line of puberty the race towards adulthood, by this third phase of the adolescent transition, is almost won.

The meta-theories and theoretical frameworks described in this chapter can help inform our understanding of pubertal and adolescent development, and enable us to be more sensitive in our professional work with young people. However, it is important to consider that each of these theoretical stances have their own particular strengths and weaknesses; and they should therefore be seen as 'partial' (academic) insights which can nevertheless guide our professional practices in working with adolescents in home, school or community settings.

---

## Applications

### 1. Measuring physical maturity
An accurate assessment of pubertal stage by physical examination is relatively easy to obtain by health professionals. If a physical examination is not practically or ethically possible, however, a good estimate can be obtained from non-invasive self-ratings and self-report scales completed by adolescents themselves or their parents.

### 2. Working with adolescents
For professionals in health care, psychology, social and community work or as educators of various kinds, two major implications emerge from the considerations of puberty and adolescence in this chapter. Firstly, as we move from biological to psychosocial interests in assessing young people's pubertal maturity the measures to be employed are at once less direct and invasive and yet more subjective and perhaps slightly less precise.

Secondly, theories of adolescence and adolescent development presented in this chapter should be regarded as an academic 'cognitive map', which can be (mentally) 'opened' to enable reflective professionals to select an appropriate theoretical approach with which to inform their professional practices in relation to working with adolescents.

---

## Further reading

Brannen, J., Dodd, K., Oakley, A. and Storey, P. (1994). *Young People, Health and Family Life.* Milton Keynes: Open University Press.

Coleman, J. C. and Hendry, L. B. (1990). *The Nature of Adolescence.* London and New York: Routledge.

Hendry, L. B., Shucksmith, J., Love, J. and Glendinning, A. (1993). *Young People's Leisure and Lifestyles.* London and New York: Routledge.

Hendry, L. B., Shucksmith, J. and Philip, K. (1995). *Educating for Health: School and Community Approaches with Adolescents.* London: Cassell.

Moore, S. and Rosenthal, D. (1993). *Sexuality in Adolescence.* London and New York: Routledge.

Plant, M. and Plant, M. (1992). *Risk-Takers: Alcohol, Drugs, Sex and Youth.* London and New York: Tavistock/Routledge.

Woodroffe, C., Glickman, M., Barker, M. and Power, C. (1993). *Children, Teenagers and Health: The Key Data.* Milton Keynes: Open University Press.

## References

Bakken, L. and Romig, C. (1992). Interpersonal needs in middle adolescents: companionship, leadership and intimacy. *Journal of Adolescence*, **15**, 3, 301–16.

Bancroft, J. (1990). The impact of socio-cultural influences on adolescent sexual development: further considerations. In *Adolescence and Puberty* (J. Bancroft and J. M. Reinisch, eds). Oxford: Oxford University Press.

Blos, P. (1962). *On Adolescence*. New York: Free Press.

Blos, P. (1967). *The Second Individuation Process of Adolescence: The Psychoanalytic Study of the Child. XXII*. New York: International University Press.

Brake, M. (1985). *Comparative Youth Sub-Cultures*. London: Routledge and Kegan Paul.

Brooks-Gunn, J. (1987). Pubertal processes and girls' psychological adaptation. In *Biological–Psychosocial Interactions in Early Adolescence: A Lifespan Perspective* (R. Lerner and T. T. Foch, eds), pp. 123–53. Hillsdale, NJ: Lawrence Erlbaum Associates.

Brooks-Gunn, J., Warren, M., Rosso, J. and Gargiuld, J. (1987). Validity of self-report measures of girls' pubertal status. *Child Development*, **58**, 829–41.

Brooks-Gunn, J. and Zahaykevich, M. (1989). Parent–child relationships in early adolescence: a developmental perspective. In *Family Systems and Life-Span Development* (K. Kreppner and R. M. Lerner, eds), pp. 223–46. Hillsdale, NJ: Lawrence Erlbaum Associates.

Bruch, H. (1985). Four decades of eating disorders. In *Handbook of Psychotherapy for Anorexia Nervosa and Bulimia* (D. M. Garner and P. E. Garfinkel, eds), pp. 7–18. New York: Guildford Press.

Bruchon-Schweitzer, M. (1990). *Une Psychologie du Corps*. Paris: P.U.F.

Clarke, A. E. and Ruble, D. N. (1978). Young adolescents' beliefs concerning menstruation. *Child Development*, **49**, 231–4.

Clausen, J. A. (1975). The social meaning of differential physical and sexual maturation. In *Adolescence in the Life Cycle* (S. Dragastin and G. Elder, eds). New York: John Wiley.

Clifford, E. (1971). Body satisfaction in adolescence. *Percept. Motor Skills*, **33**, 119–25.

Coffield, F., Borrill, C. and Marshall, S. (1986). *Growing Up at the Margins*. Milton Keynes: Open University Press.

Coleman, J. C. (1979). *The School Years*. London: Methuen.

Coleman, J. C. and Coleman, E. Z. (1984). Adolescent attitudes to authority. *Journal of Adolescence*, **7**, 131–41.

Coleman, J. C. and Hendry, L. B. (1990). *The Nature of Adolescence*. 2nd edn, London: Routledge.

Collins, W. A. (1990). Parent–child relationships in the transition to adolescence: continuity and change in interaction, affect, and cognition. In *Advances in Adolescent Development 2: From Childhood to Adolescence: A Transitional Period?* (R. Montemayor, G. Adams and T. Gullotta, eds) pp. 85–106. Newbury Park, CA: Sage.

Crisp, A. H. (1980). *Anorexia Nervosa: Let Me Be*. London: Plenum Press.

Crockett, L. J. and Petersen, A. C. (1987). Pubertal status and psychological development: findings from the early adolescence study. In *Biological and Psycho-Social Interactions in Early Adolescence: A Lifespan Perspective* (R. M. Lerner and T. T. Foch, eds) Hillsdale, NJ: Lawrence Erlbaum Associates.

Davies, E. and Furnham, A. (1986). Body satisfaction in adolescent girls. *British Journal of Medical Psychology*, **59**, 279–87.

Davis, J. (1990). *Youth and the Condition of Britain: Images of Adolescent Conflict*. London: Athlone Press.

Delaney, J., Lupton, M. J. and Toth, E. (1988) *The Curse: A Cultural History of Menstruation*. Rev. edn, Illinois: University of Illinois Press.

Demirjian, A. (1980). Dental development: a measure of physical maturity. In *Human Physical Growth and Maturation Methodologies and Factors* (F. E. Johnston, A. F. Roche and C. Susanne, eds). New York: Plenum Press.

Duncan, P. D., Ritter, P. L., Dornbusch, S. M., Gross, R. T. and Carlsmith, J. M. (1985). The effects of pubertal timing on body-image, school behaviour and deviance. *Journal of Youth and Adolescence*, **14**, 227–35.

Eagly, A. H., Ashmore, R. D., Makhijani, M. G. and Longo, L. C. (1991). What is beautiful is good, but... a meta-analytic review of research on the physical attractiveness stereotype. *Psychological Bulletin*, **110**, 109–28.

Eccles, J. S. and Midgley, C. (1989). Stage/environment fit: developmentally appropriate classrooms for early adolescents. In *Research on Motivation in Education*, **3**, (R. E. Ames and C. Ames, eds) pp. 139–86. San Diego, CA: Academic Press.

Erikson, E. (1968). *Identity: Youth and Crisis*. New York: Norton.

Eveleth, P. and Tanner, J. M. (1977). *Worldwide Variation in Human Growth*. Cambridge: Cambridge University Press.

Fallon, A. E. and Rozin, P. (1985). Sex differences in perceptions of desirable body shape. *Journal of Abnormal Psychology*, **94**, 102–5.

Faust, M. (1960). Developmental maturity as a determinant in prestige of adolescent girls. *Child Development*, **31**, 173–84.

Fend, H. (1990). Ego-strength development and pattern of social relationships. In *Coping and Self-Concept in Adolescence* (H. A. Bosma and A. E. Jackson, eds). Heidelberg: Springer-Verlag.

Fox, G. L. (1981). The family's role in adolescent sexual behaviour. In *Teenage Pregnancy in a Family Context: Implications for Policy* (T. Doms, ed.) pp. 73–130. Philadelphia: Temple University Press.

Gilligan, C. (1990). Teaching Shakespeare's sister: notes from the underground of female adolescence, Preface to *Making Connections: the Relational Worlds of Adolescent Girls at Emma Willard School* (C. Gilligan, N. P. Lyons and T. J. Hammer, eds) Cambridge, MA; Harvard University Press.

Goffman, E. (1971). *The Presentation of Self in Everyday Life*. Harmondsworth: Pelican.

Goldman, R. J. and Goldman, J. (1982). *Children's Sexual Thinking*. London: Routledge.

Greenfeld, D., Quinlan, D. M., Harding, P., Glass, E. and Bliss, A. (1987). Eating behaviour in an adolescent population. *International Journal of Eating Disorders*, **6**, 99–111.

Hampson, J. and Money, J. (1955). Idiopathic sexual precocity. *Psychosomatic Medicine*, **17**, 1–35.

Havighurst, R. J. (1972). *Developmental Tasks and Education*. 3rd edn, New York: McKay.

Hendry, L. B. (1983). *Growing Up and Going Out*. Aberdeen: Aberdeen University Press.

Hendry, L. B. (1993). Learning the new three Rs?: educating young people for modern society. *Aberdeen University Review*, **189**, Spring, 33–51.

Hendry, L. B., Shucksmith, J., Love, J. G. and Glendinning, A. (1993). *Young People's Leisure and Lifestyles*. London: Routledge.

Hendry, L. B., Shucksmith, J., Philip, K. and Jones, L. (1991). Working with young people on drugs and HIV in Grampian Region. Report of a research project for Grampian Health Board, University of Aberdeen, Department of Education.

Hsu, L. K. G. and Holder, D. (1986). Bulimia nervosa: treatment and short term outcome. *Psychological Medicine*, **16**, 6570.

Inhelder, B. and Piaget, J. (1958). *The Growth of Logical Thinking from Childhood to Adolescence*. London: Routledge and Kegan Paul.

Katchadourian, H. (1977). *The Biology of Adolescence*. San Francisco: Freeman.

Kohlberg, L. (1969). Stage and sequence: the cognitive developmental approach to socialisation. In *Handbook of Socialisation Theory and Research* (D. Goslin, ed.) Chicago: Rand McNally.

Lacey, J. H. (1983). Bulimia nervosa, binge eating and psycho-genetic vomiting: a controlled treatment study and long-term outcome. *British Medical Journal*, **286**, 1609–13.

Laufer, M. and Laufer, M. E. (1985). *Adolescence and Developmental Breakdown*. New Haven: Yale University Press.

Ledoux, S., Choquet, M. and Flament, M. (1991). Eating disorders among adolescents in an unselected French population. *International Journal of Eating Disorders*, **10**, 81–9.

Lerner, R. M. (1985). Adolescent maturational changes and psychosocial development: a dynamic interactional perspective. *Journal of Youth and Adolescence*, **14**, 355–72.

Lerner, R. M. and Karabenick, S. (1974). Physical attractiveness, body attitudes and self-concept in late adolescents. *Journal of Youth and Adolescence*, **3**, 7–16.

Livson, N. and McNeill, D. (1962). The accuracy of recalled age of menarche. *Human Biology*, **34**, 218–21.

Lloyd, M. A. (1985). *Adolescence*. London: Harper and Row.

Magnusson, D., Stattin, H. and Allen, V. L. (1985). Biological maturation and social development. A longitudinal study of some adjustment processes from mid-adolescence to adulthood. *Journal of Youth and Adolescence*, **14**, 267–83.

Marshall, W. A. and Tanner, J. M. (1969). Variations in the pattern of pubertal changes in girls. *Archives of Disease in Childhood*, **44**, 291–303.

Marshall, W. A. and Tanner, J. M. (1970). Variations in the pattern of pubertal changes in boys. *Archives of Disease in Childhood*, **45**, 13–23.

Meeus, W. (1989). Parental and peer support in adolescence. In *The Social World of Adolescents* (K. Hurrelman and U. Engel, eds). Berlin: de Gruyter.

Mussen, P. H. and Jones, M. C. (1957). Self conceptions, motivations and interpersonal attitudes of late- and early-maturing boys. *Child Development*, **28**, 243–56.

Nottelmann, E. D., Susman, E. J., Inoff-Germain, G., Cutler, G. B. Jnr., Loriaux, D. L. and Chrousos, G. P. (1987). Developmental processes in early adolescence: relations between adolescent adjustment problems and chronologic age, pubertal stage, and puberty-related serum hormone levels. *Journal of Pediatrics*, **110**, 473–80.

Offer, D. (1969). *The Psychological World of the Teenager: a Study of Normal Adolescent Boys.* New York: Basic Books.

Offer, D. and Offer, J. B. (1975). *From Teenage to Young Manhood.* New York: Basic Books.

Paikoff, R. L. and Brooks-Gunn, J. (1990). Physiological processes: what role do they play during the transition to adolescence? In *Advances in Adolescent Development: 2 From Childhood to Adolescence: a Transitional Period?* (R. Montemayor, G. Adams and T. Gullotta, eds) pp. 63–81, Newbury Park, CA: Sage.

Palmer, R., Oppenheimer, R., Dignon, A., Chalones, D. and Howells, K. (1990). Childhood sexual experience with adults. Reported by women with eating disorders. *The British Journal of Psychiatry*, **156**, 699–703.

Palmonari, A., Pombeni, M. L. and Kirchler, E. (1989). Peer groups and the evolution of the self-esteem in adolescence. *European Journal of Psychology of Education*, **4**, 3–15.

Peskin, H. (1973). Influence of the developmental schedule of puberty on learning and ego functioning. *Journal of Youth and Adolescence*, **2**, 273–90.

Petersen, A. C. (1988). *Coping with Adolescence: it's depressing!* Keynote address at an interdisciplinary research conference: Adolescent stress, social relationships and mental health. University of Massachusetts, Boston.

Petersen, A. C. and Crockett, L. J. (1985). Pubertal timing and grade effects on adjustment. *Journal of Youth and Adolescence*, **14**, 191–206.

Petersen, A. C., Crockett, L., Richards, M. and Boxer, A. (1988). A self report measure of pubertal status: reliability, validity and initial norms. *Journal of Youth and Adolescence*, **17**, 117–34.

Roche, A. F., Wainer, H. and Thissen, D. (1975). *Skeletal Maturity: The Knee Joint as a Biological Indicator.* New York: Plenum Press.

Rodriguez-Tomé, H. (1972). Le moi et l'autre dans la conscience de l'adolescent. Neuchâtel: Delachaux et Niestlé.

Rodriguez-Tomé, H. and Bariaud, F. (1990). Anxiety in adolescence: sources and reactions. In *Coping and Self-Concept in Adolescence* (H. A. Bosma and A. E. Jackson, eds). Heidelberg: Springer-Verlag.

Rosenberg, M. (1979). *Conceiving the Self.* New York: Basic Books.

Ruble, D. N. and Brooks-Gunn, J. (1982). The experience of menarche. *Child Development*, **53**, 1557–66.

Silbereisen, R. K. and Noack, P. (1990). Adolescents' orientations for development. In *Coping and Self-Concept in Adolescence* (H. A. Bosma and A. E. Jackson, eds) pp. 111–27. Heidelberg: Springer-Verlag.

Simmons, R. G. and Blyth, D. A. (1987). *Moving into Adolescence: The Impact of Pubertal Change and School Context.* New York: Aldine de Gruyter.

Simmons, R. G., Blyth, D. A. and McKinney, K. L. (1983). The social and psychological effects of puberty on white females. In *Girls at Puberty: Biological and Psychosocial Perspectives* (J. Brooks-Gunn and A. Petersen, eds). New York: Plenum.

Simmons, R. and Rosenberg, S. (1975). Sex roles and self image. *Journal of Youth and Adolescence*, **4**, 229–56.

Stattin, H. and Magnusson, D. (1990). *Pubertal Maturation in Female Development*. Hillsdale, NJ: Lawrence Earlbaum Associates.

Steinberg, L. D. (1987). The impact of puberty on family relations: effects of pubertal status and pubertal timing. *Developmental Psychology*, **23**, 451–60.

Stoltzman, S. M. (1986). Menstrual attitudes, beliefs and symptoms. Experiences of adolescent females, their peers, and their mothers. *Journal of Healthcare for Women International*, **7**, 97–114.

Streitmatter, J. L. (1985). Cross-sectional investigation of adolescent perceptions of gender roles. *Journal of Adolescence*, **8**, 183–93.

Tanner, J. M. (1962). *Growth at Adolescence*. 2nd edn, Oxford: Blackwell.

Tanner, J. M. (1978). *Foetus into Man*. London: Open Books.

Teja, J. S. (1976). Single case study. Periodic psychosis of puberty: a longitudinal case study. *Journal of Nervous and Mental Disease*, **162**, No. 1.

Tiggemann, M. and Pennington, B. (1990). The development of gender differences in body-size dissatisfaction. *Australian Psychologist*, **25**, 306–13.

Tobin-Richards, M. H., Boxer, A. M. and Petersen, A. (1983). The psychological significance of pubertal change: sex differences in perceptions of self during early adolescence. In *Girls at Puberty: Biological and Psychosocial Perspectives* (J. Brooks-Gunn and A. Petersen, eds) New York: Plenum.

Youniss, J. and Smollar, J. (1985). *Adolescent Relations with Mothers, Fathers and Friends*. Chicago IL: University of Chicago Press.

Youniss, J. and Smollar, J. (1990). Self through relationship development. In *Coping and Self-Concept in Adolescence* (H. A. Bosma and A. E. Jackson, eds). Heidelberg: Springer-Verlag.

# 3

# Menstruation and the premenstrual syndrome

Anne Walker

Menstruation has been associated with women's reproductive capacity for centuries, although the biological connection between ovulation and menstruation was only established in the late nineteenth century. The folklore and literature of ancient cultures portrays menstruation as mysterious, connecting women with the moon or supernatural forces, for good or ill. Accounts of menstruation in relatively modern cultures generally portray it as a potentially debilitating or malevolent force. In recent years, premenstrual syndrome (PMS or PMT) has been described as evidence that premenopausal women, like adolescents, are subject to the vagaries of 'raging hormones'. In this chapter, Anne Walker considers the experience of menstruation and the research evidence which has investigated the assumed link between menstruation and psychological well-being. Is menstruation a disease which drives women mad once a month – or is our experience and interpretation of menstruation influenced by the negative stereotypes which surround it?

> *Oh! menstruating woman, thou' rt a fiend*
> *From whom all nature should be closely screened.*
>
> Old saying

> *...the monthly trauma of menstruation, which in many cases can lead to wildly irrational behaviour...*
>
> The Mail on Sunday, 4 April 1993

If folklore and recent press reports are to be believed, menstruation is a source of great debility to women, and trauma to society. Every month, under the influence of this malevolent force, women become irrational, angry and vengeful, creating havoc at home and at work, murderous at worst and indecisive at best.

The aim of this chapter is to investigate the truth of this 'Jekyll and Hyde' stereotype. Do women really become murderous and irrational before and during menstruation? If so, is this all women or just some women? Every month or just some months? How and why might menstruation make women mad? Or are we simply imagining this menstrual madness?

I will begin by describing menstruation, and outlining the beliefs and practices which surround it. I will then go on to discuss the feelings and experiences which women report around menstruation, and to evaluate the different theories which have developed to explain these feelings.

## What is menstruation?

Menstruation is the term used to describe a discharge of blood and fluid from the womb through the vagina, which occurs amongst adult women at approximately monthly intervals between the ages of about 13 (see Chapter 2) and 50 (see Chapter 4). Menstrual fluid consists of blood and tissue from the wall of the uterus. The amount of fluid lost can vary from one period to the next, and from one woman to the next, so estimates of the 'heaviness' of periods are very subjective (Baldwin, Whalley and Pritchard, 1961). Studies which have collected used towels and tampons and measured blood and tissue loss estimate that women lose on average 40 ml of each during menstruation (Golub, 1992).

The time interval between two episodes of menstruation (the menstrual cycle) is usually counted from the first day of bleeding, and varies both between women and over time. It is often assumed that menstruation occurs regularly, every 28 days; in fact only about 1 in 8 cycles is exactly this length (Treloar, Boynton, Behn and Brown, 1967; Vollman, 1977; Voda, Morgan, Root and Smith, 1991; Munster, Schmidt and Helm, 1992), and cycle lengths can vary dramatically. For example, an average length of 35 days has been found amongst young teenage women, reducing to a minimum of 27 days amongst women in their early forties and then increasing to 52 days amongst women in their mid-fifties (Vollman, 1977).

The length of menstrual bleeding is also variable, and uterine bleeding can occur 'between' periods, e.g. midcycle bleeding or 'breakthrough' bleeding during oral contraceptive use. Some women experience 'spotting' or 'staining' in the days before the full period begins, or after the main flow is past. Defining the beginning and end of menstruation is not as straightforward as it sounds, neither is defining what is menstruation and what is not (Snowden, 1977; Snowden and Christian, 1983).

The purpose of menstruation remains a mystery. Folk theories of menstruation suggest that menstruation purifies or cleanses the body, releasing the tainted blood which builds up during the month. Most of the women in an interview study by Snow and Johnson (1977) said that menstruation rids the system of impurities which might otherwise cause illness or poison the system. Religious theories of menstruation similarly have tended to emphasize the impurity of menstruation, suggesting either that it occurs to punish women for an original sin (i.e. Eve's temptation of Adam), or that it occurs because women are periodically possessed by supernatural deities (Weideger, 1985). Religions based on moon-worship are more positive about menstruation, seeing it as a connection between the human and spiritual world, a magical and powerful force (Shuttle and Redgrove, 1978). Modern scientific theories of menstruation suggest that it has no purpose, occurring only as a by-product of an inefficient reproductive system. It is a waste product with no functional use, representing only the woman's failure to achieve pregnancy (Martin, 1989; Laws, 1990). So, whilst some 'folk' theories suggest that frequent menstruation is healthy and natural, most 'medical' theories suggest that frequent menstruation is unnatural and even harmful (e.g. Dennis, 1992).

An alternative theory has been proposed recently by Margie Profet (1993). She suggests that menstruation (and other forms of uterine bleeding) protect the uterus and reproductive system from pathogens carried by sperm. Hence, regular menstruation is a valuable and natural function, quite independent of ovulation, which protects the female reproductive system from infection. Whilst this more positive view of menstruation requires further examination, it does explain some important observations which other hypotheses cannot. For example, uterine bleeding as the first sign of infection, higher rates of vaginal and uterine infections amongst women who are not menstruating regularly, and so on. Perhaps the 'folk' theories of menstruation as a cleansing process are more accurate than is commonly thought.

## Attitudes towards and expectations of menstruation

*Each time I have a period ... I have the feeling that in spite of all the pain, unpleasantness and nastiness, I have a sweet secret ... that is why, although it is nothing but a nuisance to me in a way, I shall always long for the time that I shall feel that secret within me again.*

Anne Frank, 1953

This extract from Anne Frank's diary reminds us that menstruation is a subjective experience, and, in our culture, a private and usually hidden one. The ambivalence she expresses is found too in empirical studies of women's attitudes.

Five major attitudes towards menstruation have been identified by Brooks-Gunn and Ruble (1980), and embodied in the Menstrual Attitudes Questionnaire, which has been widely used (Brooks-Gunn and Ruble, 1986; Stoltzman, 1986; Olasov-Rothbaum and Jackson, 1990; Dye, 1991). This research suggests that menstruation can be seen as a natural event, a means for women to keep in touch with their bodies; a debilitating event, causing pain or unpleasant symptoms; a predictable event which can be anticipated; a bothersome event which women just have to put up with; or a non-event which has no effect on women.

All of these factors are endorsed by young American women, hence menstruation is seen as a predictable and bothersome event, as well as a debilitating one, and one which can be positive by keeping them in touch with their bodies. Men and pre-adolescent girls rate menstruation as more debilitating and having a greater effect on mood than women (Clarke and Ruble, 1978; Brooks-Gunn and Ruble, 1986), suggesting that cultural stereotypes exaggerate actual experiences.

A qualitative study based on interviews with a wide age range of menstruating women in London revealed three broad categories of attitude which they call 'acceptance', 'fatalism' and 'antipathy' (Scambler and Scambler, 1985; 1993). Women who showed acceptance (25%) saw periods as a normal part of life and non-problematic. Some of this group expressed positive feelings about menstruation, referring to it as healthy or feminine. The fatalism group (27%) viewed periods as a 'necessary evil' – unpleasant but unavoidable. The 'antipathy' group (48%) expressed unconditional negative views of menstruation, ranging from mild dislike to hostility. These views appear to be similar to those of the younger women surveyed in previous studies. They may also be influenced by symptom experience, since a higher proportion of women in the 'antipathy' group reported high levels of menstrual distress (Scambler and Scambler, 1985).

These mixed feelings about menstruation can also be identified in the everyday language and medical terminology which is used to describe it (Ernster, 1975; Shuttle and Redgrove, 1978; Delaney, Lupton and Toth, 1988; Martin, 1989; Laws, 1990; Golub, 1992). Some common terms are listed in Table 3.1, reflecting positive, negative and neutral feelings about menstruation. Hence,

**Table 3.1** Some menstrual expressions

*American women (from Golub, 1992)*

| | | |
|---|---|---|
| Period | Monthlies | That time of the month |
| Those days | Old faithful | The Moon |
| I've got my friend | Aunt Tilly is here | George is visiting |
| My redheaded friend | Somebody's visiting | Got the Grannies |
| The curse | Unwell | Sick time |
| I've got the misery | Under the weather | Cramps |
| Weeping womb | Wrong time of the month | Monthly troubles |
| I'm indisposed | I fell off the roof | The nuisance |
| The plague | Package of troubles | Riding a white horse |
| Riding the cotton pony | Plug is in | White cylinder week |
| On the rag | Back in the saddle | Cotton bicycle |
| The red flag is up | Celebrating | Red letter day |
| Safe again | This is my day | Mother Nature's gift |
| I've got my flowers | The benefit | Woman's friend |
| Too wet to plough | Flying Baker | Can't go swimming |
| Tide's in | Tide's out | Red light |
| Ice-boxed | Cherry in Sherry | Covering the Waterfront |
| Beno (There'll be no fun) | | |

*British women (from Laws, 1990)*

| | | |
|---|---|---|
| Has it come? | That time of the month | The friend |
| Lady in the red dress | I've got a visitor | Monthlies |
| Are you on? | Unwell/ill | Issue |
| Jam and bread | Grandma's here | Aunt Susie |
| The reds are in | Are you seeing red? | Poorly |
| Curse | Redlight | The red flag's flying |
| The captain's aboard | Star period | United's playing at home today |

*Men (from Ernster, 1975; Laws, 1990)*

| | | |
|---|---|---|
| Jam rags | Jammy rags | Jam sandwich |
| Jam roll | Having the rags up | On the rag |

menstruation may be welcomed as a sign of non-pregnancy, a symbol of femininity or health and normality, or it may be described in neutral terms as a visitor or time-related event. Negative terms usually imply sexual unavailability or associated pain and discomfort. Many of these terms suggest disgust or a feeling that menstruation is dirty. Even the terms 'sanitary protection' and 'feminine hygiene', to describe towels and tampons, imply that menstruation is unhygienic and that the world should be protected from it (McNeill, 1992; Berg and Block-Coutts, 1994).

Men's attitudes, as judged by the terms they use for menstruation, are almost entirely negative, referring usually to menstrual paraphernalia or presumed sexual non-availability (Laws, 1990; Ernster, 1975). They are also used differently, as terms of abuse towards other men, and in jokes rather than as direct references to menstruation and women (Laws, 1990).

It is not surprising, given these negative attitudes, that both men and women expect menstruation to have adverse effects. In particular menstruation is expected to have a detrimental effect on moods and intellectual abilities (Koeske and Koeske, 1975; Parlee, 1974; Walker, 1992a). These stereotypical beliefs are important because they influence not only the observations women themselves make about menstruation, but also the questions researchers ask, as we shall see in the next section.

# Experiences of menstruation

*... its approach is generally preceded by certain feelings of oppression or deviation from the ordinary state of health, which warn the individual of what is to happen. There is in particular, a sensation of fulness about the lower part of the belly and of relaxation about the uterine system.*

Hamilton, 1813

*It astonishes me how much better I feel once my period has arrived. The physical symptoms may be worse perhaps with backache and fatigue particularly for the first three days, but at least the irrational anger and distorted and depressed view of reality evaporates.*

Respondent to *Woman* magazine survey, quoted in Walker (1988)

Changes in physical and emotional well-being associated with menstruation have long been reported. Early reports suggested that women not only feel differently during menstruation, but also experience sensations or changes in well-being which signal the onset of menstruation, but are these supported by empirical research?

Studies in this area can be divided into two broad categories. Those which ask women to recall how they felt before, during, and sometimes after, a recent or 'typical' menstrual period (retrospective studies) and those which ask women to rate themselves on predetermined measures of well-being frequently (usually daily) over one or more menstrual cycles (prospective studies). Prospective studies are now considered the 'gold standard' of menstrual cycle research since Mary Parlee demonstrated the existence of stereotypical responses to retrospective questionnaires (Parlee, 1974). Almost invariably these studies require women to rate themselves on measures devised by the researcher and hence they tend to be biased towards the measurement of negative moods and experiences (influenced by the stereotypes of the researchers). An additional quirk of the literature is that researchers have focused on the days before menstruation rather than menstruation itself, although the precise length of the premenstrual phase studied varies dramatically from 2 to 14 days (Fausto-Sterling, 1992).

## Retrospective studies

A wide variety of physical and emotional premenstrual and menstrual experiences are reported by women in retrospective surveys. Moos (1969) identified 150 separate menstrual 'symptoms', and Sophie Laws (1985) collated a list of ninety-five physical or emotional complaints from the medical literature. These range from 'transient nymphomania' to 'suicide'; from 'headache' to 'feelings of worthlessness'. Abdominal pain, nausea and faintness tend to be associated with menstruation rather than the days before the onset of bleeding. Positive experiences have also been reported. Logue and Moos (1988) have suggested that 5–15 per cent of women experience increased excitement, energy and well-being around menstruation. Reports also exist of increased activity, improved performance on some tasks and heightened sexuality. So, almost any human state, good, bad or indifferent has been reported to occur around menstruation (see Table 3.2). Are these just random occurrences, or are they associated with menstruation?

**Table 3.2** Diagnostic criteria for 'late luteal phase dysphoric disorder'

A.  In most menstrual cycles during the past year, symptoms in (B) occurred during the last week of the luteal phase and remitted within a few days after onset of the follicular phase.

B.  At least five of the following symptoms have been present for most of the time during each symptomatic late luteal phase, at least one of the symptoms being either (1), (2), (3) or (4):
    (1)  marked affective lability
    (2)  persistent and marked anger or irritability
    (3)  marked anxiety or tension
    (4)  markedly depressed mood
    (5)  decreased interest in usual activities
    (6)  easy fatiguability or marked lack of energy
    (7)  subjective sense of difficulty in concentrating
    (8)  marked change in appetite, overeating or specific food cravings
    (9)  hypersomnia or insomnia
    (10) other physical symptoms, such as breast tenderness or swelling, headaches, joint or muscle pain, a sensation of 'bloating' and weight gain.

C.  The disturbance seriously interferes with work or with usual social activities or relationships with others.

D.  The disturbance is not merely an exacerbation of the symptoms of another disorder.

E.  Criteria are confirmed by prospective daily self-ratings during at least two symptomatic cycles.

*Source*: DSM-III-R, American Psychiatric Association (1987)

This question can only really be addressed in prospective studies (see below). Researchers using retrospective techniques have however looked for a unifying factor amongst the variety of symptoms reported which might suggest a non-random process.

An example of this type of research is a study by John Richardson (1989). He gave a list of forty-four frequently reported premenstrual symptoms to 217 undergraduate women students and asked them to indicate which, if any, they regularly experienced premenstrually. The thirty-six most frequently reported symptoms were subjected to factor analysis, from which six factors emerged:

- **cognitive impairment**: including items on poor work or academic performance, lowered efficiency or judgement
- **emotionality**: irritability, mood swings, crying, tension, depression, anxiety
- **faintness**: dizziness, faintness, nausea, hot flushes
- **social impairment**: avoiding social activities
- **behavioural impairment**: poor coordination, confusion
- **fluid retention**: weight gain, swelling.

In addition to these, many women reported breast pain around menstruation, but this was not associated with any of the other symptoms. A second order factor analysis suggested the existence of a single over-arching factor, linking together all of the separate single clusters (except breast pain). This type of analysis suggests that there is a unifying factor between these experiences, and that they may be menstrually related. Breast pain may also be menstrually related, but is not linked to anything else. However, this type of retrospective analysis is crucially flawed because of the possibility that women are reporting stereotypes rather than 'real' experiences, or because experiences around menstruation are remembered more easily than at other times of the month. We may simply be measuring a unified stereotype here, rather than a real phenomenon.

**Prospective studies**

The only way to investigate whether the experiences women report really do occur more frequently around menstruation than at other times is to study women prospectively, i.e. to obtain frequent reports of moods and feelings. This type of study requires highly motivated participants, willing to complete often lengthy questionnaires or cognitive tests regularly (often every day) for at least six weeks (ideally studies should be much longer than this). Consequently, such studies are usually small and involve either students or women complaining of severe symptoms.

Prospective studies of cognitive performance began with Leta Hollingworth's pioneering work in the early years of this century (Hollingworth, 1914), and are still conducted today. A wide variety of different cognitive measures have been used, with different numbers of women and over different time periods. However, despite this variability between studies the outcomes are fairly consistent. Most studies suggest that women on average perform just as well academically or on cognitive tests before or during menstruation as they do at any other time (Sommer, 1978; Sommer, 1992). Indeed performance on some tests may be enhanced premenstrually (Dye, 1992).

Studies of physical state are equally consistent, but with the opposite conclusion. Some physical experiences are more likely to occur during menstruation than at any other time. Abdominal pain and feelings of bloatedness, for instance, are significantly more frequent during menstruation than at other times (Asso, 1983). Breast pain too is closely associated with menstruation (Walker, 1994; Mansel, Preece and Hughes, 1980).

Studies of mood during the menstrual cycle are less consistent. Several studies have shown slight but not statistically significant deteriorations in mood premenstrually (Wilcoxon, Schrader and Sherif, 1976; Slade, 1984). These have usually been relatively small (twenty to thirty participants) and composed of young women students. Larger samples, for statistical reasons, are more likely to reveal significant phase effects (Gannon, 1985), and non-student samples studied prospectively are more likely to show significant cyclical fluctuations in mood, being least happy and most irritable around menstruation (Walker and Bancroft, 1990).

A problem with this type of research is that average findings are usually reported. These may not reflect the experience of any of the women in the sample, and implicitly assume that all women have the same type of premenstrual or menstrual experiences. In a recently reported study, I have shown that premenstrual emotional experiences vary widely both between women and across cycles in individual women (Walker, 1994). For example, although this study showed an overall increase in depression and irritability premenstrually, this was not true for all of the participants. In one cycle, 13 per cent of this sample felt happier before menstruation than afterwards, while 45 per cent were less happy premenstrually than postmenstrually. Similarly with irritability scores, 17 per cent were less irritable premenstrually than postmenstrually, while 53 per cent showed the expected premenstrual increase. The overall averages had obscured some women's positive experiences. A comparison across two consecutive cycles also suggested that one premenstrual phase is not necessarily predictable from the last. Only 6.6 per cent of the variance in pre and postmenstrual mood change scores in a second cycle could be accounted for by knowing comparable ratings from the first.

**Conclusions**

It would seem, then, that women may experience any number of emotional and mood states around menstruation, some of which are welcome and some of which we might prefer to be without. On average these states are not debilitating and the link between them and menstruation is unclear. Physical experiences such as pain and swelling are clearly related to menstruation, but emotional and cognitive experiences do not show such a close association.

So, why do we continue to believe that women are emotionally upset around menstruation, and why are such feelings reported with such frequency in retrospective accounts? This may be because menstruation is itself memorable. Remembering our last period triggers our recall of events and experiences around that time, while similar events at other times are forgotten. Alternatively, we may be conditioned to report our feelings in a stereotypical way (even prospectively). It may be that 'real' changes in mood or intellectual abilities are compensated for and not reported in daily diaries or revealed in psychological tests. Variability between cycles could account for differences between retrospective and prospective accounts, as noted above. Perhaps the use of an illness metaphor and terms like 'symptoms' obscures changes which are more subtle and not perceived by women as signs of illness, just sensations which accompany or precede menstruation. Perhaps menstruation is a relatively trivial influence on women's day-to-day emotional or cognitive state and its effects are obscured in prospective studies by the effects of other events. Women may report a connection retrospectively because we are aware of our own history of experience and are able to 'factor out' menstrual cycle effects from other effects in our daily lives. In other words, prospective studies need to ask women why they think they feel a certain way on a particular day, not just how they feel. A final alternative is that the symptoms listed on retrospective questionnaires are experienced regularly by women, but they are not related to menstruation. Women may be endorsing the symptoms on such questionnaires and acknowledging that they are not present all the time, inferring that they are menstrually related because this is the connection the researcher has made.

Clearly, despite some lengthy and time-consuming research, our understanding of the psychological aspects of menstruation for most women is severely limited – arguably because the questions asked about it have been so limited.


# The premenstrual syndrome

Premenstrual syndrome (PMS) is a scientific construct which has proved difficult to define or diagnose (Condon, 1993). As noted earlier, there are many historical references to a connection between emotional tension or changes in mood and the time around menstruation, although these sources do not usually discriminate between menstruation itself and the days before menstruation (Richardson, 1992). It was not until the twentieth century, however, that severe tension premenstrually was identified as an abnormality or dysfunction in the medical literature (Frank, 1931; Horney, 1931). These clinicians are referring to a condition of extreme and debilitating tension and anxiety in the days before menstruation, which is relieved at menstrual onset.

Medical and popular concern with premenstrual tension was fairly minimal until the publication of a paper in the *British Medical Journal* in 1953 by Raymond Greene and Katharina Dalton. This paper broadened the concept of premenstrual tension, and renamed women's experiences premenstrual syndrome to encompass any severe emotional or physical symptoms occurring before menstruation. Dalton has defined PMS as 'any symptoms or complaints which regularly occur just before or during early menstruation but are absent at other times of the cycle' (Dalton, 1977). This broad definition, lacking any criterion of symptom severity, has resulted in estimates of widespread prevalence of PMS (e.g. Pennington, 1957, estimated 95 per cent prevalence of PMS), and concerns about the pathologization of women (e.g. Laws, 1985).

Throughout the 1980s considerable research effort was expended in an attempt to precisely define and diagnose severe PMS, distinguishing a debilitating menstrually related disorder (albeit with a wide variety of potential symptoms), from the 'normal' menstrual experiences described above. Most of these new definitions arose within psychiatry (rather than gynaecology) and emphasize premenstrual depression and irritability rather than physical symptoms – hence the development of new names – late luteal phase dysphoric disorder (LLPDD) or premenstrual dysphoric disorder (PMDD). Most clinical studies have used the diagnostic criteria outlined in the *American Diagnostic and Statistical Manual of Mental Disorders* (DSM) (American Psychiatric Association, 1987), and these are outlined in Table 3.2.

Studies which use this type of criterion suggest that between 3 and 5 per cent of women regularly experience debilitating premenstrual symptoms (Andersch, Wendestam, Hahn and Ohman, 1986). A recent carefully designed epidemiological study of 6232 women aged 20–49 found no evidence of a widespread premenstrual dysphoric disorder and estimated the risk of clinically significant affective symptoms attributable to the premenstrual state at 1 per cent (Ramcharan, Love, Fick and Goldfien, 1992). It is worth noting that 4–6 per cent of the sample were rating negative effect symptoms as severe at all phases of the cycle, suggesting that the distress women report is real even if the connection with menstruation is unclear.

Considerable confusion remains, however, about the concept of PMS. It is not clear whether PMS represents the extreme of a continuum of experience, i.e. having PMS is analogous to being taller than average (Walker, 1988), or a disease state which is either present or absent, i.e. having PMS is analogous to having measles (Ramcharan, Love, Fick and Goldfien, 1992). Neither is it clear whether there is a single premenstrual syndrome (Jorgensen, Rossignol and Bonnlander, 1993) or several premenstrual syndromes (Abraham, 1983). Additionally prospective ratings often fail to confirm a clear link between the severe distress which clinic attenders may call PMS and menstruation (Yuk, Jugdutt, Cumming et al., 1990), suggesting a multiplicity of causal mechanisms. The DSM definition is difficult to implement (Gallant, Popiel, Hoffman et al., 1992) and is not universally accepted (Caplan, McCurdy-Myers and Gans, 1992). In addition, it is a consensus definition constructed by biomedical researchers and clinicians and imposed on the experiences women report, rather than a definition based on epidemiological or descriptive studies.

# Explanations for menstrual experiences

Explanations for menstrual experiences and PMS[1] deriving from most schools of thought from psychoanalytic to sociobiological can be found in the literature. Some of these explanations have been more popular than others, and the amount of research from different perspectives varies greatly. The biomedical perspective has been both the most popular and the most widely researched. In this chapter, I will restrict discussion to four of the major paradigmatic approaches to PMS, the biomedical, psychosomatic, psychological and social constructionist approaches, and will conclude by introducing a fifth, the biopsychosocial approach.

## The biomedical approach

Biomedical research assumes that abnormal experiences are the result of identifiable diseases with their origins in physiological dysfunction (Engel, 1977). Hence the first step in research is to define abnormality and diagnose a disease state, whilst the second step is the identification of a consistently associated physiological dysfunction.

In PMS research, this approach is exemplified in Robert Frank's paper in 1931. Firstly, women who complain of 'indescribable tension from ten to seven days preceding menstruation' (Frank, 1931) are defined as abnormal, and secondly the cause of the abnormality is attributed to a physiological process, in this case an assumed abnormal and excessive secretion of the female sex hormones. The major 'female' hormones, oestrogen and progesterone, were identified in the 1920s, hence it is not surprising that a link was suggested at this time (Norris, 1987). In this model, premenstrual experiences are only considered abnormal if they are severe and interfering with daily life. Non-debilitating experiences are acknowledged and are attributed (by implication) to normal hormonal fluctuations. It is only the abnormal state which requires explanation and research.

In the absence of a clear, consistent and meaningful definition, studies of potential physiological mechanisms are difficult to interpret and it is probably not surprising that most reviews of this extensive literature remain inconclusive (Walker, 1992b; Parry and Rausch, 1988). Studies of relationships between premenstrual symptoms and ovarian hormones can demonstrate clear temporal links – symptoms occur in the second half of the cycle, although they are not dependent on ovulation (Walker and Bancroft, 1990). Associations between hormone levels or other measures and symptom severity have not been demonstrated however. It seems likely that endogenous mood rhythms and neuroendocrine systems are involved in some way but the details of such mechanisms remain obscure (Dinan and O'Keane, 1991). It may be that neuroendocrine and uterine or ovarian systems interact to produce specific symptom clusters (Bancroft, Williamson, Warner et al., 1993).

[1] NB: the term PMS is being used here to refer to severe and debilitating premenstrual experiences, affecting a small number of women in a significant proportion of their menstrual cycles.

## The psychosomatic model

In this model, too, non-debilitating premenstrual experiences are attributed to 'normal' hormonal fluctuations. Women who experience severe premenstrual distress, however, are hypothesized to differ psychologically rather than physiologically from asymptomatic women. The woman's temperament or psychology causes an exacerbation of the normal premenstrual experience through a psychosomatic mechanism.

Within this paradigm the psychological mechanisms which have been investigated include intrapsychic conflicts (Horney, 1931), conflict about or denial of femininity (Levitt and Lubin, 1967; Berry and McGuire, 1972), personality characteristics (Coppen and Kessel, 1963), and responses to stress (Woods, 1986).

Studies of personality characteristics have identified significant differences between sufferers and non-sufferers of PMS, or significant associations between the degree of symptom reported and personality variables. For example, Coppen and Kessel (1963) found significant correlations between PMS and neuroticism in a sample of 465 women. Some important criticisms of these studies have been made by Linda Gannon (1985). She points out, for example, that studies have generally failed to distinguish between menstrual and premenstrual symptoms, that personality measures and PMS questionnaires are often confounded, that multiple hypotheses are tested allowing possibly spurious correlations to arise, and that the reported correlations are small (although significant) suggesting that psychological characteristics at best may account for less than 5 per cent of the variance in menstrual distress scores (or vice versa).

The final caution in addition to these must be the remainder that all the studies are correlational and cannot therefore demonstrate causal links, only associations.

It seems then that whilst there is some evidence that personality characteristics like neuroticism and anxiety-proneness may be associated with PMS, the nature of the association is unclear and the degree of association is very small. As these characteristics have been associated with symptom reporting in a wide variety of physical conditions (Watson and Pennebaker, 1989), it is unlikely that this association is a specific causal mechanism.

A similar story can be told for studies which have interpreted links between menstrual disorders and conflict about or denial of femininity. Here the results are contradictory, with some studies suggesting that women with PMS do feel more resentment of traditional role expectations (May, 1976; Berry and McGuire, 1972), while others suggest the opposite, i.e. that women reporting menstrual distress are more traditionally feminine (Gough, 1975). However, the cautions about correlational studies and interpretation of findings apply equally.

The psychosomatic approach then has yielded fairly inconclusive findings. There is no evidence from these studies to suggest an exclusive or even dominant psychogenic aetiology for PMS. However, the small associations which have been found suggest that psychological factors may be involved, either as cause, consequence or both.

## The psychological approach

The biomedical and psychosomatic approaches both consider menstrual experiences from the point of view of abnormality. They are concerned predominantly with the alleviation of distress amongst women who are complaining of it. These explanations imply causal mechanisms for non-debilitating premenstrual experiences, almost by default, but they are not concerned with explaining those experiences.

The psychological approach criticizes these on three grounds. First, the attempt to understand normality from the study only of abnormality; second, the emphasis only on the premenstrual phase of the menstrual cycle; and, third, the failure to consider the diversity of women's experiences, for example the occurrence of positive feelings premenstrually, and the variability in experiences between cycles. The biomedical and psychosomatic models are fundamentally too simplistic to account for women's experiences.

The psychological approach places menstruation and the premenstrual days in the context of a continuous menstrual cycle (Asso, 1983, 1992), one example of the many cycles and rhythms which influence men's and women's lives (e.g. circadian rhythms, circannual rhythms). Not only do ovarian hormones fluctuate during the cycle, so does almost every other physiological and neurophysiological process. In particular the cycle is characterized by fluctuations in central nervous system activity, or arousal. Most of the time, these arousal levels pre-dispose women to positive feelings and behaviour. After ovulation, however, the situation is more complex, as Asso (1992) writes:

> Premenstrually, several factors can (but do not always) together contribute to a fairly negative background climate. In addition to low central nervous system arousal and often high autonomic activation, there is activity of other neurophysiological variables, such as monoamine oxidase and endorphin; there may be fluid retention, skin problems, and so on; there is the influence of complex cognitive processes, which can include memory of past discomfort, over-concentration on changes, and attitudes to the whole cycle which can affect the experience of the premenstrual phase.

Hence, the feelings that a woman experiences premenstrually depend not only on her ovarian hormone levels, nor even on the changes in arousal which these are associated with, but also on her physical state, her memories of past experiences, and her beliefs and attitudes about menstruation. This model predicts, and therefore explains, variability both between and within women.

A social cognition dimension of this model applies the classic research by Schachter and Singer (1962) and others on the social construction of emotions to premenstrual symptoms (Ruble and Brooks-Gunn, 1979; Rodin, 1976). It is argued that states of arousal are themselves neutral, but become labelled as happiness or anger or irritability, etc., depending on the attributions made by the person experiencing them. These attributions depend on the cultural beliefs and stereotypes of the individual and their social context. The negative beliefs about menstruation in western societies may lead individuals to develop negative expectations about the premenstrual phase, and hence to label autonomic activity at this time as negative rather than positive (e.g. restlessness rather than creative energy). Individual differences are hypothesized to arise from differences in the strength of negative expectations, which may themselves be related to socialization, attitudes towards femininity, and so on; and/or differences in the degree of cyclical change in arousal.

There is plenty of evidence that cultural stereotypes and expectations exist (e.g. Walker, 1992a). Cyclical changes in arousal have also been identified

(Asso, 1992). Some supporting evidence also comes from cross-cultural studies, which suggest that women in non-westernized cultures do not complain of premenstrual changes (Snowden and Christian, 1983), however, these studies are limited by language use. It is possible that symptoms exist but are not defined as a problem, and therefore not reported to the researcher (McNeill, 1992).

Studies directly linking the degree of symptom experience with strength of attitudes and cyclical arousal are lacking. However, there is some evidence to suggest that women attribute negative experiences to menstruation (Koeske and Koeske, 1975), and that this attribution is socially acceptable (Brooks-Gunn and Ruble, 1986; Walker, 1993). These findings suggest that social cognition processes are involved in the definition of a physical (or emotional) state as a symptom and the subsequent reporting of that symptom to a clinician, as has been shown in other contexts (e.g. Pennebaker, 1981; Pennebaker and Epstein, 1983). However, the role of psychological processes or cyclical changes in arousal in the genesis of these physical and emotional states is as yet unknown.

### The social construction model

Whilst all of the other approaches accept the dysfunctional and, implicitly, pathological nature of PMS, the social construction approach disputes this. It is acknowledged that women may experience distress, which can be severe for some women on some occasions. However, these are side effects of normal physiological processes and not the result of pathology. The definition of this distress as pathological is culturally constructed (see Laws, 1985; Rome, 1986; Martin, 1989; Rodin, 1992).

Evidence in support of the social constructionist argument is derived from analysis of medical and popular texts, historical documents and everyday discourse, rather than measurement of symptoms or delineation of syndromes. Ample evidence can be found in historical studies (especially of the nineteenth century) of the tendency to medicalize and pathologize women's behaviour (Ehrenreich and English, 1973; Ussher, 1989, 1991, 1992a and b; Showalter, 1985). Women are often described as inherently weak, sickly or irrational, and as having abnormalities in comparison to men which are attributed to their reproductive capacity. This view is summarized by a physician writing in 1870, who said: '[it is] as if the Almighty, in creating the female sex, had taken the uterus and built up a woman around it' (quoted in Smith-Rosenberg and Rosenberg, 1973). Uterine activities such as menstruation were considered particularly detrimental (Cayleff, 1992; Bullough and Voght, 1973; Wood, 1973–74; Showalter and Showalter, 1970).

Echoes of this can be found in more recent medical and popular literature about PMS (Rome, 1986; Laws, 1985; Rittenhouse, 1991; Rodin, 1992). In particular, the press coverage of two murder trials in which PMS was cited as a mitigating factor provoked much concern about the immutable and biologically determined unreliability of women (Holtzmann, 1988; Laws, 1985), despite the vastly greater incidence of antisocial behaviour amongst men.

The definition of cyclical changes in well-being as pathological is implied in the diagnosis of PMS and perpetuates the notion of women as incomplete or dysfunctional men. Hence, the diagnoses are socially constructed and should not be the concern of the medical profession (Rodin, 1992). That is not to say that distress occurring premenstrually (or at any other time) should be ignored or left untreated – simply that it should not necessarily be attributed to a pathological state. The realities of many women's lives offer a more meaningful explanation for the distress which is reported.

This approach too can be criticized. Whilst it may be true that PMS is socially constructed, this is true of all medical diagnoses. As Dingwall (1992) points out:

> There are no diseases in nature, merely relationships between organisms. Diseases are produced by conceptual schemes imposed on the natural world by human beings, which value some states of the body and disvalue others.

The application of this argument is important in political terms since it exposes medicine as an agent of social control (Laws, 1985), however it offers little in terms of understanding why women experience distress or intervening to relieve distress (Ussher, 1992a).


## Conclusions: a biopsychosocial approach to the menstrual cycle

In this chapter we have seen that menstruation is surrounded by myth, taboo and ambivalence. Menstruation is part of a rhythm with biological, psychological and physical associations. Although we know very little about the nature of this rhythm or the feelings which women experience throughout the cycle, we know a lot about how women feel in the few days before menstruation.

We have seen that the biomedical approach to research has described the changes which occur, and has found associations between some physiological measures and some symptom measures. However, defining a syndrome of severe premenstrual symptoms has proved more difficult than expected and, as yet, no clear physiological difference has been found between women, or cycles, with severe premenstrual symptoms and those without. The psychosomatic approach has similarly proved unsuccessful. Although personality characteristics are associated with menstrual distress, the association is small and its aetiological significance cannot be tested. The psychological approach has suggested that cyclical arousal and attributional processes may be important in symptom perception and reporting, but no evidence has yet been found to link the occurrence of physical or emotional states premenstrually with attitudes, attributions or arousal. The social construction approach has reminded us of the cultural beliefs about women and menstruation and the dangers of pathologization and medicalization of menstrual experiences, however it has not offered a means for further understanding or relieving women's distress.

Where does that leave us? It would appear that menstrual cycle experiences are neither wholly biologically determined nor wholly psychosomatic. Cultural and personal beliefs and attributions are of significance. Physical and emotional experiences may interact (Jarvis and McCabe, 1991). In addition, there are discrepancies between the number of women experiencing distress and the number complaining of it (Scambler and Scambler, 1993; Metcalf, Livesey, Wells and Braiden, 1989), suggesting that psychological processes of symptom perception and attribution are of significance (Pennebaker, 1981).

In many areas of health care, the biomedical model is no longer the most useful conceptual tool, and a biopsychosocial approach may be of more benefit (Engel, 1977). Biopsychosocial models attempt to reconcile biological factors with psychological and sociocultural mechanisms, without giving one precedence over the others. These models imply that symptoms are multiply determined, and may have different origins in different people. Hence, treatment strategies should be individualized, based on individual symptom experience and individual circumstance. Whilst this philosophy probably reflects the practice of clinicians treating women who complain of PMS (O'Brien, 1987; Robertson, 1991), it is not the philosophy which underpins most research studies.

Multivariate and biopsychosocial models have been proposed in relation to PMS (Alberts and Alberts, 1990; Miota, Yahle and Bartz, 1991; Ussher 1992b) and other 'reproductive syndromes' (Hunter, 1993, and see Chapter 4), which hold promise for future research developments. These models develop and formalize the psychological approach to menstrual experiences described earlier. Physiological, psychological and sociocultural factors are seen to interact both in symptom timing (i.e. around menstruation) and symptom severity. The identification of these feelings and sensations as symptoms is seen to depend on beliefs and attributions together with personal and cultural models of illness. Hence, the processes of symptom perception, illness identification and help-seeking behaviour are similar to those in other physical conditions (Murray, 1990; Scambler and Scambler, 1985). Symptom perception may result in symptom reporting to a medical (or other) practitioner if lay referral networks support this and clinicians are perceived to offer an efficacious solution. These processes may themselves arouse confirmation-seeking self-monitoring activities, increasing the expectation effects which previous studies have noted (e.g. Olasov and Jackson, 1987).

Menstrual cycle research to date has been heavily influenced by cultural notions of gender (see Chapter 1), and misogynistic views of femininity. As Laws (1990) points out, most of the explanations for the negative experiences reported by women imply that women themselves are to blame for their pain or distress. Either because we have faulty biology, or because we have faulty personalities or over-active imaginations. It is to be hoped that biopsychosocial models will encourage researchers and clinicians to think of the menstrual cycle as only one of the many factors which influence women's lives and well-being – a force which is present, but not necessarily dominant. More importantly, new insights are unlikely unless research and practice is based on women's experiences rather than cultural stereotypes.

## Applications

### 1. Sympton prevention

Negative attitudes towards and stereotypes of menstruation associate a normal process with illness and pathology. Discussion of positive or neutral aspects is important to minimize excessive medicalization of menstruation.

On a psychological level, enhancing self-esteem and self-awareness may encourage appropriate symptom attribution, and hence appropriate intervention strategies.

### 2. Symptom management

If distress is experienced around menstruation, a holistic approach is needed to management considering the women's life circumstances, her beliefs and attitudes towards menstruation as well as her physical symptoms and hormonal state. Psychological interventions, such as the development of coping skills and relaxation training may be useful for pain and stress management.

Healthy eating and appropriate exercise may act at a physiological level as well as a psychological one to reduce symptoms or help women to cope. Many remedies have been recommended for severe PMS, although women vary in which they find most useful. Prescribed remedies in conjunction with counselling and psychological intervention may be the most appropriate.

## Further reading

Golub, S. (1992). *Periods: From Menarche to Menopause.* Newbury Park, CA: Sage.

Richardson, J. T. E. (ed.) (1992). *Cognition and the Menstrual Cycle.* New York, Springer-Verlag.

Scambler, A. and Scambler, G. (1993). *Menstrual Disorders.* London: Tavistock/Routledge.

Warner, P. and Walker, A. (eds) (1992). *The Menstrual Cycle,* special issue of the *Journal of Reproductive and Infant Psychology,* **10** (2), 63–128.

## References

Abraham, G. (1983). Premenstrual tension. *Journal of Reproductive Medicine,* **28,** 433–4.

Alberts, P. S. and Alberts, M. S. (1990). Unvalidated treatment of premenstrual syndrome. *International Journal of Mental Health,* **19,** 69–80.

American Psychiatric Association (1987). *Diagnostic and Statistical Manual of Mental Disorders-III-R.* Washington DC: American Psychiatric Association.

Andersch, B., Wendestam, C., Hahn, L. and Ohman, R. (1986). Premenstrual complaints I: Prevalence of premenstrual symptoms in a Swedish urban population. *Journal of Psychosomatic Obstetrics and Gynaecology,* **5,** 39–50.

Asso, D. (1983). *The Real Menstrual Cycle*. Chichester: John Wiley.

Asso, D. (1992). A reappraisal of the normal menstrual cycle. *Journal of Reproductive and Infant Psychology*, **10**, 103–10.

Baldwin, R., Whalley, P. and Pritchard, J. (1961). Measurements of menstrual blood loss. *American Journal of Obstetrics and Gynecology*, **81**, 739–42.

Bancroft, J., Williamson, L., Warner, P., Rennie, D. and Smith, S. (1993). Perimenstrual complaints in women complaining of PMS, menorrhagia, and dysmenorrhea: Toward a dismantling of the premenstrual syndrome. *Psychosomatic Medicine*, **55**, 133–45.

Berg, D. H. and Block-Coutts, L. (1994). The extended curse: being a woman every day. *Health Care for Women International*, **15**, 11–22.

Berry, C. and McGuire, F. L. (1972). Menstrual distress and acceptance of sexual role. *American Journal of Obstetrics and Gynecology*, **114**, 83–7.

Brooks, J., Ruble, D. and Clark, A. (1977). College women's attitudes expectations concerning menstrual-related changes. *Psychosomatic Medicine*, **39**, 288–97.

Brooks-Gunn, J. and Ruble, D. (1980). The menstrual attitude questionnaire. *Psychosomatic Medicine*, **42**, 503–12.

Brooks-Gunn, J. and Ruble, D. (1986). Men's and women's attitudes and beliefs about the menstrual cycle. *Sex Roles*, **14**, 287–99.

Bullough, V. and Voght, M. (1973). Women, menstruation and nineteenth century medicine. *Bulletin of the History of Medicine*, **47**, 66–82.

Caplan, P., McCurdy-Myers, J. and Gans, M. (1992). Should 'premenstrual syndrome' be called a psychiatric abnormality? *Feminism and Psychology*, **2**, 27–44.

Cayleff, S. E. (1992). She was rendered incapacitated by menstrual difficulties: Historical perspectives on perceived intellectual and physiological impairment among menstruating women. In *Menstrual Health in Women's Lives* (A. J. Dan and L. L. Lewis, eds). Urbana: University of Illinois Press.

Clarke, A. E. and Ruble, D. N. (1978). Young adolescents' beliefs concerning menstruation. *Child Development*, **49**, 231–4.

Condon, J. T. (1993). Investigation of the reliability and factor structure of a questionnaire for assessment of the premenstrual syndrome. *Journal of Psychosomatic Research*, **37**, 543–51.

Coppen, A. and Kessel, N. (1963). Menstruation and personality. *British Journal of Psychiatry*, **109**, 711–21.

Dalton, K. (1977). *The Premenstrual Syndrome and Progesterone Therapy*. London: Heinemann.

Delaney, J., Lupton, M. J. and Toth, E. (1988). *The Curse: A Cultural History of Menstruation*. Revised edn. Urbana: University of Illinois Press.

Dennis, R. (1992). Cultural change and the reproductive cycle. *Social Science and Medicine*, **34**, 485–9.

Dinan, T. G. and O'Keane, V. (1991). The premenstrual syndrome: a psychoneuroendocrine perspective. *Ballieres Clinical Endocrinology and Metabolism*, **5**, 143–65.

Dingwall, R. (1992). 'Don't mind him – he's from Barcelona': qualitative methods in health studies. In *Researching Health Care: Designs, Dilemmas, Disciplines* (J. Daly, I. McDonald and E. Willis, eds). London: Routledge.

Dye, L. (in press). Attitudes to and experience of menstruation in a German University sample. *Proceedings of the 1991 Conference of the Society for Menstrual Cycle Research*, Hamilton Cross, Seattle, USA.

Dye, L. (1992). Visual information processing and the menstrual cycle. In *Cognition and the Menstrual Cycle* (J. Richardson, ed.) New York: Springer-Verlag.

Ehrenreich, B. and English, D. (1973). *Complaints and Disorders: The Sexual Politics of Sickness*. London: Writers and Readers Publishing Co-operative.

Engel, G. L. (1977). The need for a new medical model. *Science*, **196**, 129–36.

Ernster, V. (1975). American menstrual expressions. *Sex Roles*, **1**, 1–13.

Fausto-Sterling, A. (1992). *Myths of Gender: Biological Theories about Women and Men*. Revised edn. New York: Basic Books.

Frank, A. (1953). *The Diary of a Young Girl*. New York: Basic Books.

Frank, R. T. (1931). The hormonal causes of premenstrual tension. *Archives of Neurology and Psychiatry*, **26**, 1053–7.

Gallant, S. J., Popiel, D. A., Hoffman, D. M., Chakraborty, P. K. and Hamilton, J. (1992). Using daily ratings to confirm premenstrual syndrome/late luteal phase dysphoric disorder. Part II. What makes a real difference? *Psychosomatic Medicine*, **54**, 167–81.

Gannon, L. (1985). *Menstrual Disorders and Menopause: Biological, Psychological and Cultural Research*. New York: Praeger.

Golub, S. (1992). *Periods: From Menarche to Menopause*. Newbury Park, CA: Sage.

Gough, H. G. (1975). Personality factors related to reported severity of menstrual distress. *Journal of Abnormal Psychology*, **84**, 59–65.

Graham, C. and McGrew, W. (1992). Social factors and menstrual synchrony in a population of nurses. In *Menstrual Health in Women's Lives* (A. J. Dan and L. L. Lewis, eds). Urbana: University of Illinois Press.

Greene, R. and Dalton, K. (1953). The premenstrual syndrome. *British Medical Journal*, **1**, 1007–14.

Hamilton, A. (1813). *A Treatise on the Management of Female Complaints*. Peter Hill: Edinburgh.

Hollingworth, L. S. (1914). Functional periodicity: An experimental study of the mental and motor abilities of women during menstruation. New York, Teachers College, Columbia University. *Contributions to Education*, **69**, 86–101.

Holtzman, E. (1988). Premenstrual syndrome as a legal defense. In *The Premenstrual Syndromes* (L. H. Gise, ed.). New York: Churchill Livingstone.

Horney, K. (1931). Die prämenstruellen Verstimmungen. *Zeitschrift für Psychanalytische Pädagogik*, **5**, 161–7.

Hunter, M. (1994). *Counselling in Obstetrics and Gynaecology*. Leicester: British Psychological Society.

Jarvis, T. and McCabe, M. (1991). Women's experience of the menstrual cycle. *Journal of Psychosomatic Research*, **35**, 651–60.

Jorgensen, J., Rossignol, A. M. and Bonnlander, H. (1993). Evidence against multiple premenstrual syndromes: results of a multivariate profile analysis of premenstrual symptomatology. *Journal of Psychosomatic Research*, **37**, 257–63.

Koeske, R. K. and Koeske, G. F. (1975). An attributional approach to mood and the menstrual cycle. *Journal of Personality and Social Psychology*, **31**, 473–8.

Laws, S. (1985). Who needs PMT? A feminist approach to the politics of premenstrual tension. In *Seeing Red: The Politics of Pre-Menstrual Tension* (S. Laws, V. Hey and A. Eagan, eds). London: Hutchinson.

Laws, S. (1990). *Issues of Blood: The Politics of Menstruation*. London: Macmillan.

Laws, S. (1992). It's just the monthlies, she'll get over it: menstrual problems and men's attitudes. *Journal of Reproductive and Infant Psychology*, **10**, 117–28.

Levitt, E. E. and Lubin, B. (1967). Some personality factors associated with menstrual complaints and menstrual attitudes. *Journal of Psychosomatic Research*, **11**, 267–70.

Logue, C. M. and Moos, R. H. (1988). Positive perimenstrual changes: toward a new perspective on the menstrual cycle. *Journal of Psychosomatic Research*, **32**, 31–40.

McNeill, E. (1992). Variations in subjective state over the oral contraceptive pill cycle: the influence of endogeneous steroids and temporal manipulations. University of Edinburgh: unpublished PhD thesis.

Mansel, R., Preece, P. and Hughes, L. (1980). Treatment of cyclical breast pain with bromocriptine. *Scottish Medical Journal*, **25**, S65–70.

Martin, E. (1989). *The Woman in the Body: A Cultural Analysis of Reproduction*. Milton Keynes: Open University Press.

May, R. R. (1976). Mood shifts and the menstrual cycle. *Journal of Psychosomatic Research*, **20**, 125–30.

Metcalf, M. G., Livesey, J. H., Wells, J. E. and Braiden, V. (1989). Mood cyclicity in women with and without the premenstrual syndrome. *Journal of Psychosomatic Research*, **33**, 407–18.

Miota, P., Yahle, M. and Bartz, C. (1991). Premenstrual syndrome: A bio-psycho-social approach to treatment. In *Menstruation, Health and Illness* (D. Taylor and N. Woods, eds) pp. 143–51. New York: Hemisphere.

Moos, R. H. (1969). Typology of menstrual cycle symptoms. *American Journal of Obstetrics and Gynaecology*, **103**, 390–402.

Munster, K., Schmidt, L. and Helm, P. (1992). Length and variation in the menstrual cycle – a cross-sectional study from a Danish county. *British Journal of Obstetrics and Gynaecology*, **99**, 422–9.

Murray, M. (1990). Lay representations of illness. In *Current Developments in Health Psychology* (P. Bennett, J. Weinman and P. Spurgeon, eds) London: Harwood Academic Press.

Norris, R. (1987). Historical development of progesterone therapy. In *Premenstrual Syndrome* (B. Ginsburg and B. Carter, eds). New York: Plenum Press.

O'Brien, P. M. S. (1987). *Premenstrual Syndrome*. Oxford: Blackwell Scientific Publications.

Olasov, B. and Jackson, J. (1987). Effects of expectancies on women's reports of moods during the menstrual cycle. *Psychosomatic Medicine*, **49**, 65–78.

Olasov-Rothbaum, B. and Jackson, J. (1990). Religious influence on menstrual attitudes and symptoms. *Women and Health*, **16**, 63–78.

Parlee, M. B. (1974). Stereotypic beliefs about menstruation. A methodological note on the Moos MDQ and some new data. *Psychosomatic Medicine*, **36**, 229–40.

Parry, B. L. and Rausch, J. L. (1988). Evaluation of biologic research. In *The Premenstrual Syndromes* (L. D. Gise, ed.) pp. 47–58.

Pennebaker, J. W. (1981). *The Psychology of Physical Symptoms*. New York: Springer-Verlag.

Pennebaker, J. W. and Epstein, D. (1983). Implicit psychophysiology: effects of common beliefs and idosyncratic physiological responses on symptom reporting. *Journal of Personality*, **51**, 468–96.

Pennington, V. M. (1957). Meprobamate (Miltown) in premenstrual tension. *Journal of the American Medical Association*, **164**, 638–41.

Profet, M. (1993). Menstruation as a defense against pathogens transported by sperm. *Quarterly Review of Biology*, **68**, 335–86.

Ramcharan, S., Love, E., Fick, G. and Goldfien, A. (1992). The epidemiology of premenstrual symptoms in a population-based sample of 2650 urban women: attributable risk and risk factors. *Journal of Clinical Epidemiology*, **45**, 377–92.

Richardson, J. T. E. (1989). Student learning and the menstrual cycle: premenstrual symptoms and approaches to studying. *Educational Psychology*, **9**, 215–38.

Richardson, J. T. E. (1992). *Cognition and the Menstrual Cycle*. New York: Springer-Verlag.

Rittenhouse, C. A. (1991). The emergence of premenstrual syndrome as a social problem. *Social Problems*, **38**, 412–25.

Robertson, M. (1991). A survey of multidimensional and interdisciplinary approaches to pre-menstrual syndrome. In *Menstruation, Health and Illness* (D. Taylor and N. Woods, eds) pp. 129–43. New York: Hemisphere.

Rodin, J. (1976). Menstruation, reattribution and competence. *Journal of Personality and Social Psychology*, **33**, 345–53.

Rodin, M. (1992). The social construction of premenstrual syndrome. *Social Science and Medicine*, **35**, 49–56.

Rome, E. (1986). Premenstrual syndrome examined through a feminist lens. *Health Care for Women International*, **7**, 145–52.

Ruble, D. and Brooks-Gunn, J. (1979). Menstrual symptoms: a social cognition analysis. *Journal of Behavioural Medicine*, **2**, 171–94.

Scambler, A. and Scambler, G. (1985). Menstrual symptoms, attitudes and consulting behaviour. *Social Science and Medicine*, **20**, 1065–8.

Scambler, A. and Scambler, G. (1993). *Menstrual Disorders*. London: Tavistock/Routledge.

Schachter, S. and Singer, J. (1962). Cognitive, social and psychological determinants of emotional state. *Psychological Review*, **69**, 379–99.

Showalter, E. (1985). *The Female Malady: Women, Madness and English Culture, 1830–1980*. New York: Pantheon Books.

Showalter, E. and Showalter, E. (1970). Victorian women and menstruation. *Victorian Studies*, **14**, 83–9.

Shuttle, P. and Redgrove, P. (1978). *The Wise Wound: Menstruation and Everywoman*. London: Victor Gollancz.

Slade, P. (1984). Premenstrual emotional changes in normal women: fact or fiction? *Journal of Psychosomatic Research*, **28**, 1–7.

Smith-Rosenberg, C. and Rosenberg, C. (1973). The female animal: medical and biological views of woman and her role in the nineteenth century. *Journal of American History*, **60**, 332–56.

Snow, L. and Johnson, S. (1977). Modern day menstrual folklore. *Journal of the American Medical Association*, **237**, 2736–9.

Snowden, R. (1977). The statistical analysis of menstrual bleeding patterns. *Journal of Biosocial Science*, **9**, 107–20.

Snowden, R. and Christian, B. (1983). *Patterns and Perceptions of Menstruation*. Beckenham, Kent: Croom Helm.

Sommer, B. (1978) Stress and menstrual distress. *Journal of Human Stress*, **4**, 41–7.

Sommer, B. (1992). Cognitive performance and the menstrual cycle. In *Cognition and the Menstrual Cycle* (J. T. E. Richardson, ed.) pp. 39–66. New York: Springer-Verlag.

Stoltzman, S. M. (1986). Menstrual attitudes, beliefs and symptom experiences of adolescent females, their peers and their mothers. *Health Care for Women International*, **7**, 96–114.

Treloar, A., Boynton, R., Behn, B. and Brown, B. (1967). Variation of the human menstrual cycle through reproductive life. *International Journal of Fertility*, **12**, 77–126.

Ussher, J. (1989). *The Psychology of the Female Body*. London: Routledge.

Ussher, J. (1991). *Women's Madness: Misogyny or Mental Illness*. London: Harvester Wheatsheaf.

Ussher, J. (1992a). The demise of dissent and the rise of cognition in menstrual cycle research. In *Cognition and the Menstrual Cycle* (J. T. E. Richardson, ed.) pp. 132–73. New York: Springer-Verlag.

Ussher, J. (1992b). Research and theory related to female reproduction: Implications for clinical psychology. *British Journal of Clinical Psychology*, **31**, 129–51.

Voda, A. M., Morgan, J., Root, J. and Smith, K. (1991). The Tremin Trust: An intergenerational research program on events associated with women's menstrual and reproductive lives. In *Menstruation, Health and Illness* (D. Taylor and N. Woods, eds) pp. 5–18. New York: Hemisphere.

Vollman, R. F. (1977). *The Menstrual Cycle*. Philadelphia: W. B. Saunders.

Walker, A. (1988). The relationship between premenstrual symptoms and the ovarian cycle. University of Edinburgh: unpublished PhD thesis.

Walker, A. (1992a). Men's and women's beliefs about the influence of the menstrual cycle on academic performance: a preliminary study. *Journal of Applied Social Psychology*, **22**, 896–909.

Walker, A. (1992b). Premenstrual symptoms and ovarian hormones: a review. *Journal of Reproductive and Infant Psychology*, **10**, 67–82.

Walker, A. (1993). 'It's just the time of the month': the social acceptability of menstrual attributions and its significance for symptom reporting. Paper presented at British Psychological Society Scottish Branch Annual Conference, Crieff Hydro Hotel, November.

Walker, A. (1994). Mood and well-being in consecutive menstrual cycles: methodological and theoretical implications. *Psychology of Women Quarterly*, **18**, 271–89.

Walker, A. and Bancroft, J. (1990). Relationship between premenstrual symptoms and oral contraceptive use: a controlled study. *Psychosomatic Medicine*, **52**, 86–96.

Watson, D. and Pennebaker, J. W. (1989). Health complaints, stress and disease: exploring the central role of negative affectivity. *Psychological Review*, **96**, 234–54.

Weideger, P. (1985). *History's Mistress*. Harmondsworth: Penguin.

Wilcoxon, L. A., Schrader, S. L. and Sherif, C. W. (1976). Daily self reports on activities, life events and somatic changes during the menstrual cycle. *Psychosomatic Medicine*, **38**, 399–417.

Wood, A. D. (1973–74). The fashionable diseases: women's complaints and their treatment in nineteenth-century America. *Journal of Interdisciplinary History*, **4**, 25–52.

Woods, N. F. (1986). Socialization and social context: Influence on perimenstrual symptoms, disability and menstrual attitudes. *Health Care for Women International*, **7**, 115–29.

Yuk, V., Jugdutt, A., Cumming, C., Fox, E. and Cumming, D. (1990). Towards a definition of PMS: A factor analytic evaluation of premenstrual change in non-complaining women. *Journal of Psychosomatic Research*, **34**, 439–46.

# 4

# Menopause

## Myra S. Hunter

The new reproductive technologies may enable women to conceive and carry a baby after the menopause, however the last menstrual period usually marks the end of women's reproductive capacity. For most women, the menopause occurs naturally with ovarian function gradually changing over a number of years. For a smaller group, the menopause occurs suddenly and artificially following surgical removal of the ovaries and hysterectomy. Like adolescence and menstruation, the menopause has been seen as a time of raging hormonal change. Unlike menstruation and adolescence, though, the menopause is also associated with ageing. Not surprisingly, the negative stereotypes surrounding it in our culture are strong and pervasive. In this chapter, Myra Hunter considers women's experience of the menopause and asks whether 'the change' is really as unpleasant as we might expect. Is the medical view of the menopause as a 'hormone-deficiency disease' the best way of understanding women's experiences, and should all women be using hormone-replacement therapy to stay 'feminine forever'?

## Introduction

The menopause literally refers to a woman's last menstrual period. The average age of menopause is between 50 and 51 years – median 50.78 in Britain (McKinlay and Jefferys, 1974) – and the typical range is 45 to 55 years. The World Health Organisation (WHO, 1981) defines the menopause as 'permanent cessation of menstruation resulting from loss of ovarian follicular activity'. The last menstrual period is preceded by a gradual reduction in output of oestrogen by the ovaries and fewer ovulatory cycles (Richardson, 1993). In medical discourse the term climacteric has a broader, although somewhat vague, time frame from the beginning of ovarian changes to at least one year after the final menstruation.

The most commonly used classification of the menopause in clinical research and practice is to divide women into one of three stages, based on menstrual criteria (Jaszmann, 1973): (1) Premenopausal women have regular periods, i.e. no obvious change in their menstrual cycle, (2) perimenopausal women have menstruated during the past year, but have experienced irregular menstruation, while (3) postmenopausal women have not menstruated at all during the preceding year. Nevertheless, women do not necessarily progress steadily from one stage to the next (Kaufert and Gilbert, 1988). For example, some may oscillate between stages, while others might find that menstruation ceases without warning. The time taken from the first change in menstrual cycles to a year after the last cycle is, on average, four years (McKinlay et al., 1992). Menopause is considered premature if it occurs before the age of 40, and it can occur at any age as the result of disease or following surgery, such as oophorectomy (removal of the ovaries). Hormonal measures (lowered oestradiol (< 100 pm/litre) and raised follicle stimulating hormone (> 30 iu/litre)) can also be used to confirm menopausal status.

The menopause transition is characterized by hot flushes and night sweats (also called vasomotor symptoms), which are experienced by between 50 and 70 per cent of women in western cultures during the peri- and postmenopause. For the majority, these are not seen as problematic. However, it is estimated that between 10 and 15 per cent find them difficult to cope with, largely because of their frequency or their disruptive effects upon sleep.

Despite the fact that hot flushes are the only clear symptom of the menopause (Utian, 1975), a vast array of physical and emotional problems have at one time or another been attributed to it (for example, poor memory and concentration, loss of libido, irritability, anxiety, headaches, problems with skin and hair, aching limbs and joints, itchiness, weight gain, and loss of energy), and terms such as climacteric syndrome and menopausal syndrome are still commonly found in medical texts. The colloquial term for the menopause – the change of life – reflects the view that the biological menopause usually occurs during a stage of life that is typically associated with role changes, emotional and social and adaptations (Neugarten, 1979). Thus, 'the change' in popular discourse might encompass many physical, psychological and social changes which may occur during mid-life.

In summary then, the menopause (the final menstrual period) can be regarded as a marker in a more gradual process of physiological change (characterized by hormonal changes, and commonly by hot flushes), occurring concurrently with age and developmental changes, in a psychosocial and cultural context. The relative contributions of biological, psychological, social and cultural factors to a woman's experience of the menopause, and the meaning it has for her, are considered in the sections that follow. Discussion centres primarily upon explanations of psychological experiences (in particular depressed mood) – a controversial topic that has been the subject of heated debate in the past two decades (Ballinger, 1990; Hunter, 1990a; Studd and Smith, 1993), and which is paralleled by similar discussions about women's experiences of other stages of the reproductive cycle (Ussher, 1992).

## Theoretical perspectives

### The biomedical model

> Menopause, once regarded as ... a neurosis, was redefined as a deficiency disease by physicians in the 1960s, when synthetic oestrogen became widely available.
>
> McCrea, 1983

The current dominant view of the menopause is found in the biomedical literature and is based on the premise that menopause is a cluster of physical and emotional symptoms that is caused by deficiency in reproductive hormones. It follows that the symptoms should be treated by replacing the missing hormones with oestrogen, or hormone replacement therapy.

Menopausal problems were first 'treated' by doctors in eighteenth-century France (Wilbush, 1979). In the nineteenth century the developments of psychiatry, gynaecology and psychoanalysis reinforced the link between woman's emotional state and her reproductive capacity. Menopause was defined as a physiological crisis that could cause disease under certain conditions, such as non-adherence to her prescribed role. Emotional symptoms, such as expressions of anger or distress, were at times regarded as sexual or hysterical in origin, and gynaecological surgery, such as hysterectomy, performed as a cure. It was even believed that the menopause caused psychosis, termed involutional melancholia (Krafft-Ebbing, 1877).

The identification of the main hormones produced by the ovaries in the 1920s led to the development of oestrogen therapy, initially prescribed for hot flushes and night sweats: a treatment which was first used in Germany and the USA. The publication of Robert Wilson's *Feminine Forever* in the USA in 1966 had a major impact upon sales of oestrogen therapy. He conceptualized menopause as a definite disease with twenty six psychological and physical complaints that oestrogen could avert, including hot flushes, osteoporosis, vaginal atrophy, sagging and shrinking breasts, wrinkles, absentmindedness, frigidity, depression, alcoholism and even suicide. He argued that women should be treated in their thirties and continue until death in order to preserve 'total femininity'. His view of the menopause has been assimilated into mainstream gynaecological discourse, as illustrated by the following quotes (Utian, 1977; Studd and Smith, 1993):

It constitutes a true endocrine ovarian deficiency disease, equivalent, for example, to insulin deficiency in diabetes mellitus, and hence a pathological state or true metabolic disorder requiring recognition and correction.

The declining oestrogen levels of the climacteric are also thought to give rise to a variety of symptoms, collectively referred to as the climacteric syndrome, namely insomnia, depression, headaches, dyspareunia, loss of libido, generalized aches and pains, poor concentration, irritability, poor memory, anxiety and urinary frequency.

In the past twenty years hormone replacement therapy (HRT) has been advocated for longer-term health problems of older women, as well as for vasomotor symptoms which occur during the menopause transition. Longer-term use of HRT (five to ten years or more) is generally recommended for the prevention of osteoporosis (loss of bone mass in later life, resulting in fractures (Smith, 1990)), and for the prevention of cardiovascular disease (the major cause of death in the over sixties (Paganini-Hill, Ross and Henderson, 1988)). However, at the same time, there has been concern about the long-term risks of HRT, especially in relation to breast cancer, a matter which is still contentious (Brinton, 1990). Thus the boundaries of the 'disease' have shifted over time from a transitional state to a more permanent postmenopausal condition.

The biomedical model defines the menopause as a health problem, rather than a normal developmental process, and strips experiences, such as emotional distress or lack of sexual desire, of their psychosocial contexts, labelling them as symptoms. Underlying this model is the assumption that the menopause has marked salience, compared to other factors, to the health and well-being of mid-aged and older women. The model also *implies* that the menopause is to be avoided at all costs, since a host of problems might ensue if HRT is not sought.

### Sociocultural models

The menopause has been described as a Western culture-bound syndrome, reflecting a preoccupation with youth, beauty and sexuality.

Wilbush, 1979

The sociocultural model of the menopause is a social science perspective that emerged in the 1970s, partly in reaction to the biomedical view. The menopause (a biological process) is construed as a natural process having little or no effect on women; rather, menopausal symptoms are seen as cultural constructions (Kaufert, 1982). Negative stereotypes and attitudes towards menopause and ageing, as well as women's social role, and role changes, are identified as the main causes of any distress.

This model draws upon historical, anthropological and sociological studies. A woman's status is often believed to be reversed at the menopause. For example, in societies that adhere to rigid menstrual taboos, women might enjoy more personal and social freedom after the menopause. In such societies attitudes to, and experience of, the menopause would be expected to be more positive. Marsha Flint's pioneering work, comparing the experience of menopause in North America and in an Indian Rajput community, described the absence of menopausal symptoms in the Indian culture where older women gained heightened social prestige, while, in constrast, in North America there is no reward for reaching menopause (Flint, 1975).

Sociologists and psychologists have tended to emphasize role changes or psychosocial stresses in explanations of possible distress experienced by women during midlife. For example, it can be a time of adjustment to achievements and disappointments, a time when children leave home, a time to reassess long-term relationships, a time when parents might die or require care, as well as a time when ageing becomes more difficult to ignore. While a woman's position in her chronological, biological and social life cycle may be more variable than is traditionally assumed, evidence from epidemiological studies is used to support the hypothesis that concurrent, coincidental life stresses are important influences upon a woman's health and well-being during the menopause.

From both the above perspectives (focusing upon cultural attitudes and values, or social roles and stresses) biological changes are seen as having minimal impact. Instead the meaning of the menopause is socially constructed. If the menopause is seen as a traumatic time, then any distress resulting from concurrent life changes might be attributed to it, and in this way negative stereotypes are maintained.

**Psychological models**

Few psychological models have been developed. Those that have been proposed have attempted to explain individual differences in experience of the menopause and interactions between causal factors.

Two psychologists have developed theories related to the life stress hypothesis. Greene (1984) formulated the 'vulnerability model', which is a variant of Brown and Harris's (1978) life stress model, applied to midlife. Here life stresses (particularly bereavements and other losses) are seen as the main causes of distress and symptom reports. In this model 'climacteric vulnerability' is influenced by both physiological instability (hormonal) and psychosocial factors, and moderates a woman's reactions to and ability to cope with existing problems, previous problems and age-related changes. Therefore hormonal factors, as well as psychosocial factors, are thought to increase a woman's vulnerability.

An interesting interactive model has been put forward by Ballinger, Cobbin, Krivanek and Saunders (1979). The authors suggest that stress can exacerbate a woman's experience of the menopause by directly affecting her hormones (reducing oestrogen levels), in addition to having a negative impact upon her well-being in general. Ballinger draws on her own research to support this explanation.

Finally, a biopsychosocial model has been proposed (Hunter, 1994); this is outlined at the end of the next section.

## The evidence

Two main questions will be addressed in this section:

1. Are women more likely to be depressed or have emotional problems during the menopause transition?
2. To what extent do the explanatory models, described above, contribute to our understanding of a woman's experience of the menopause?

The main focus here is upon epidemiological and treatment studies. The term 'depressed mood' is used broadly to represent a continuum of self-reported depressive symptoms; reference to clinical depression or emotional well-being is indicated as necessary.

### Are women more likely to be depressed or have emotional problems during the menopause transition?

The evidence from epidemiological studies has been equivocal, hampered by both polarized theoretical views and methodological problems. The latter are described in detail by Kaufert and Gilbert (1988), and include the use of un-standardized symptom questionnaires, unclear definitions of menopausal status, generalizations from clinic samples and lack of control of age effects and cohort differences when comparisons are made between women at different stages of the menopause. The recognition of the influence of stereotyped beliefs upon perceptions of the menopause has led some researchers to take steps to prevent awareness that the menopause is the focus of study.

Of the cross-sectional studies carried out in the 1960s and 1970s, comparing pre-, peri- and postmenopausal women of different ages, some found peri-menopausal increases in the prevalence of psychological symptoms (Jaszmann, van Lith and Zaat, 1969; Bungay, Vessay and McPherson, 1980), while in other studies no changes were evident (McKinlay and Jefferys, 1974; Thompson, Hart and Durno, 1973). Several prospective studies were set up in the 1980s, using broadly similar methodologies, in Manitoba (Kaufert, Gilbert and Tate, 1992), in Massachusetts (McKinlay et al., 1992), in Pennsylvania (Matthew, Wing and Kuller, 1990), in Norway (Holte, 1992), in the Netherlands (Oldenhave, 1991) and in south east England (Hunter, 1992a). As well as providing cross-sectional data, premenopausal women were followed for between three and five years until they become peri- or postmenopausal. Thus the effects of variables, such as past emotional state, which were confounded in earlier cross-sectional studies, could be properly examined.

Using improved methodologies, for example, larger samples and standardized measures, together these studies provide fairly strong evidence that the menopause does not have a negative impact upon the mental health of the majority of mid-aged women. However, in all the studies considerable variations between women were apparent. No significant changes in psychological symptom reports were found in four of the studies (Holte, 1992; Kaufert et al., 1992; Matthews et al., 1990; McKinlay et al., 1992). Oldenhave (1991) found an increase in psychological symptoms in perimenopausal women. However, this was associated with the experience of hot flushes and night sweats. In my own study (Hunter, 1992a) there was a small but significant increase in depressed mood reported by peri- and recently postmenopausal women, assessed by the Women's Health Questionnaire (Hunter, 1992b). However, the stage of menopause explained only 2 per cent of the variation in depressed mood, compared with over 50 per cent accounted for by psychosocial factors (see next section).

Overall, these prospective studies suggest that for most women the menopause does not lead to changes in well-being or physical symptoms, apart from possible secondary effects resulting from problematic vasomotor symptoms. Nor did it adversely affect ratings of general health or health-related behaviours, such as medication intake or number of visits to the doctor (McKinlay and McKinlay, 1986; Hunter, 1992a). Similarly, there is no evidence to support the belief, prevalent in the past, that psychiatric disorder increases at the menopause (Ballinger, 1990; Gath and Iles, 1990). Moreover, the psychiatric diagnosis of involutional melancholia was deemed invalid in 1980, and was excluded from the third edition of the American Psychiatric Association's *Diagnostic and Statistical Manual*.

In contrast, when general samples of mid-aged women have been compared with those seeking medical help (from menopause clinics), the clinic attenders report much higher rates of distress and more physical and emotional problems (Ballinger, 1985; Hunter, 1988).

**To what extent do the explanatory models, described above, contribute to our understanding of a woman's experience of the menopause?**

*Cross-cultural studies*

Studies comparing the experience of the menopause in different cultures tend to reveal a diversity of experience, suggesting that the meaning ascribed to it and women's reactions to it are, in part, culturally determined. For example, the occurrence of menopausal symptoms has been reported to be low or absent in Mayan Indians (Beyenne, 1986), North Africans in Israel (Walfish, Antonovsky and Moaz, 1984), Indian Rajput Women (Flint, 1975) and in many developing countries (Payer, 1991). Lock (1980), in a cross-sectional study of Japanese women, found that those who had stopped menstruating did not report any more emotional symptoms than the women who were still menstruating. For most women it was 'konenki' (a self-defined gradual period of change associated with ageing) which was accompanied by symptomatology. It is interesting that fewer of these Japanese women reported having hot flushes when compared with North American samples (Avis, Kaufert, McKinlay and Vass, 1993).

In recent years awareness of methodological problems and difficulties in interpretation of anthropological studies has increased. For example, Wilbush (1984) has emphasized the difference in levels of questioning – between symptoms (spontaneous complaints) and subjective sensory experiences or semeions. Similarly, the extent to which symptoms reflect differences in sensations experienced or differences in linguistic labels is a problem in the interpretation of such studies. Conceptually, the assumption that new roles for women after the menopause, such as participation in male activities, are a universal measure of status gain has rightly been questioned (Beyenne, 1986). A woman's role and status changes in non-western, as in western societies, do not necessarily correlate, or depend upon, her menopausal status. In addition, Beyenne (1986) has drawn attention to the impact of environment, diet, fertility patterns and genetic differences which may contribute to the variation in menopausal experiences across cultures.

In summary, the evidence suggests that there are likely to be genuine differences in experience of the menopause between cultures, probably mediated by both sociocultural and possibly also environmental or biological factors, but also that some variation might be explained by methodological problems.

### Studies of psychosocial factors

Midlife is commonly regarded as a time of psychosocial transition and readjustment. While some women might face widowhood, an 'empty nest' and worries about elderly parents, these events are not necessarily temporally linked to the menopause, particularly now that there is greater variability in the timing of life stages.

A child leaving home is a life change which is not necessarily stressful (Krystal and Chiriboga, 1979; Glenn, 1975). The results of general population surveys suggest that those who have 'emptied their nest' are not more prone to depression, and that this event is met with relief by many couples. Rather, family problems – such as worry about health and relationships between family members, caring for sick relatives and dealing with difficult adolescents, as well as bereavements – are more common concerns (McKinlay, McKinlay and Brambrilla, 1987; Hunter, 1992a).

There is clear evidence indicating that stressful life events, in particular losses or bereavements, lead to emotional and somatic symptoms for women in general (Brown and Harris, 1978) and for women during the menopause (Greene and Cooke, 1980). Greene and Cooke carried out a detailed investigation of the impact of a range of stresses in climacteric and postmenopausal women. Stressful life events accounted for a greater proportion of the variation in psychological and somatic symptoms than did menopausal status, and it was life events including exits (people leaving the social network) that were particularly associated with symptom reports (Cooke and Greene, 1981). The majority of exits in this study were loss of parents. Ballinger's hypothesis – that life stress has a direct biochemical effect upon oestrogen levels – has not been tested fully, but has received some support. Firstly, Ballinger, Cobbin, Krivanek and Saunders (1979) found that oestrogen levels increased as depression lifted in a sample of depressed patients. Secondly, several epidemiological studies provide evidence that women who suffer from psychiatric disorder before the menopause might be more prone to vasomotor symptoms when they reach the menopause (Hallstrom, 1973; Gath, Osborn, Bungay et al., 1987). Thirdly, laboratory evidence suggests that a woman's threshold for hot flushes might be lowered when she is under stress (Swartzman, Edelberg and Kemmann, 1990). The impact of stress upon oestrogen levels, and hence vasomotor symptoms and the interactions between these variables, warrants further attention.

Studies of marital and employment status and social class have produced equivocal results, probably because these variables are complex and produce numerous interactions. In general, women who are divorced, widowed or separated are more likely to be depressed, followed by married women, with single women having fewest problems (McKinlay, McKinlay and Brambrilla, 1987; Hunter, 1992a). In the Massachusetts study, there was an interaction between years of education and marital status, the less well-educated who were divorced or separated being most prone to depressed mood. Socioeconomic status is assessed in a variety of ways. When estimated by occupation in British studies, by years of education in North American studies or by family income, working-class women generally report more symptoms of depressed mood than middle-class women (McKinlay, McKinlay and Brambrilla, 1987; Holte, 1992; Hunter, 1992a). Employment outside the home has been shown to be protective to emotional health during midlife, but interactions with other variables need to be considered. For example, in the Massachusetts study unemployed women were least healthy and full-time home-makers reported worse emotional health than employed women (Jennings, Mazaik and McKinlay, 1984).

While it is clear that psychosocial factors, such as life stresses, are associated with reduced emotional well-being, there is no convincing evidence that mid-life is more stressful than other life stages, for example, early motherhood. When the relative impact of menopausal status and psychosocial factors has been examined, psychosocial factors account for much more of the variation in depression than menopausal status (Greene and Cooke, 1980; Hunter, 1992a; Kaufert, Gilbert and Tate, 1992).

### Studies of individual differences

Not surprisingly, the main predictor of depressed mood during the menopause is having been depressed in the past (Kaufert, Gilbert and Tate, 1992; Hunter, 1992a). For some women depressed mood is chronic, while for others, for a variety of reasons, depression can be exacerbated during the menopause. Past depression accounted for 34 per cent of the variance in depressed mood reported by menopausal women in one prospective study (Hunter, 1992a).

Attitudes and beliefs about the menopause have been investigated in the context of the cultural meaning ascribed to this life stage, and in terms of the attitudes held by individuals within a particular culture. A negative stereotype of menopausal women is prevalent in western societies where the menopause is associated with decline of functions, ageing and reduced youth and beauty (Kaufert, 1982). In one of the earliest studies of attitudes towards the menopause, Neugarten and coworkers (1963) found that women individually do not hold such negative attitudes as might be expected, and that premenopausal women had more negative attitudes than women who had already experienced the menopause. Using a different approach, Boulet, Lehert and Riphagen (1985) asked a large sample of Belgian women to rate the potential impact of the menopause upon their lives. They found that the menopause was perceived as being relatively unimportant compared to other life events. Attitudes to the menopause are not one-dimensional. In a study of British women's attitudes, expectations and stereotypes, the menopause was regarded as an event which brought emotional and physical symptoms but which also brought relief from menstruation and pregnancy (Hunter, 1988).

Attitudes and beliefs about the menopause were examined in two of the prospective studies (Avis and McKinlay, 1991; Hunter, 1992a). In both studies, those women who held negative beliefs linking the menopause with psychological and physical problems were themselves more likely to report symptoms on reaching the menopause. In the prospective phase of the south east England study, stereotyped beliefs were included as possible predictors of later depression, together with other psychosocial and health variables. A stepwise regression analysis revealed that previous depression, holding negative stereotyped beliefs, together with not being employed and being working class (assessed *before* the menopause) accounted for approximately 50 per cent of the variation in depressed mood in peri- and postmenopausal women.

In summary, psychosocial factors – including life stresses, previous depression, and probably also beliefs about the menopause – play an important role in determining a woman's emotional well-being during the menopause transition. There is little support for the empty nest syndrome or the notion that single women are more at risk at this time.

**Biomedical influences: the role of oestrogen**

From the biological perspective, psychological symptoms are seen as direct or indirect consequences of decline in ovarian function. Claims have been made, first, that oestrogen should be advocated as the treatment of choice for 'menopausal depression', and second, that oestrogen might offer an additional bonus of lifting mood or increasing well-being in non-depressed, healthy women. These two claims clearly refer to different subgroups of women and appear to be underpinned by different concerns. The first may be motivated by a desire to alleviate depression – a problem which is common amongst menopausal clinic attenders (approximately 50 per cent would be considered as clinical cases). However, this claim also assumes that depression is more prevalent for women during the menopause, and that depression experienced at the menopausal has a hormonal basis. The second claim, if corroborated, could provide evidence with which to encourage women to use and adhere to hormone replacement therapy regimens. In this case oestrogen has to be regarded as a pharmacological agent which lifts mood, rather than a replacement therapy.

There are several possible mechanisms for the inferred action of oestrogen. There is support for a central nervous system activating effect of oestrogen, from animal experiments and laboratory studies (Asso, 1983). It has been proposed that oestrogen has a monoamine oxidase inhibitory effect, leading to increased noradrenalin synthesis (Klaiber, Broverman and Vogel, 1972). In addition, oestrogen might influence tryptophan (the precursor of serotonin) release; a positive correlation has been reported between total plasma oestrogen and free plasma tryptophan in postmenopausal women (Aylward, 1976). While there is some evidence in support of both possible mechanisms, a direct relationship between oestrogen levels and depressed mood has not been generally supported.

*Correlational studies*

Correlational studies of the relationship between oestrogen level and depressed mood, in general, have failed to demonstrate a significant association between depressed mood and oestrogen levels (Alder, Bancroft and Livingstone, 1992; Ballinger, Browning and Smith, 1987; Coope, 1981; Owen, Siddle, McGarrigle and Pugh, 1992). Sherwin (1988), in one of a series of studies of surgically menopausal women, did find a positive correlation between ratings of confidence and elation and oestrogen levels. However, this was true for women treated with HRT but not untreated women, suggesting a possible pharmacological effect of oestrogen. It remains possible that withdrawal of oestrogen, as opposed to oestrogen level, might precipitate depressed mood: carefully designed research is needed to test this hypothesis.

### HRT treatment studies

Studies of the effects of oestrogen therapy upon depression or psychological symptoms are often used as evidence in the debate about the aetiology of emotional problems experienced during the menopause. It is important to remember, however, that the results of treatment studies do not provide information about aetiology. Moreover, such studies are beset by methodological problems. Samples are heterogeneous (some including depressed women, others exclude those with emotional problems, some using naturally, others surgically menopausal women), and different doses and types of oestrogen regimens are used. The placebo effects are, in general, large, and few studies control for the effects of reduction in vasomotor symptoms upon mood. It is also difficult to retain the blind status in studies when oestrogen has such a marked effect on vasomotor symptoms.

The main studies are separated into those using general clinic samples, which include more women reporting depressive symptoms, and those selecting healthier, non-depressed subjects.

*General clinic samples.* Klaiber's original study of the benefits of high doses of oestrogen for severely depressed psychiatric inpatients has not yet been replicated (Klaiber, Broverman, Vogel and Korbayasti, 1979). Using menopause clinic samples, no significant improvements have been found with oestrogen compared to placebo on standardized measures, such as the Beck Depression Scale (Coope, 1981; Campbell, 1976), Hamilton Rating Scale (Thompson and Oswald, 1977), or General Health Questionnaire (Campbell, 1976), despite improvements in vasomotor symptoms. Dennerstein and colleagues (1979) did find an improvement on the Hamilton Rating Scale, after treating women who had undergone surgical menopause. Using vasomotor symptom reports as a covariate, this improvement diminished although remained significant. Some studies find improvements in psychological symptoms using non-standardized rating scales or visual analogue scales (Campbell, 1976), while others do not (Dennerstein, Burrows, Hyman and Sharpe, 1979).

A study by Montgomery, Appelby, Brincat et al. (1987) is often quoted in support of the benefits of oestrogen therapy for menopausal women. The effects of oestrogen implants (50 mg) were compared with oestrogen plus testosterone and a placebo. Despite an initial difference between oestrogen and the placebo condition at two months post implant for the perimenopausal women in the study, there were no overall significant differences between peri- or post-menopausal subgroups and the placebo group between two and four month post implantation, nor for the postmenopausal women after two months.

*Selected healthy samples*. Sherwin (1988), in one of a series of studies of surgically menopausal women, compared oestrogen plus androgen, and oestrogen alone with a group who had been untreated (average time since operation being three to four years). Significant increases in ratings of confidence and feelings of elation, but no group differences in depression were evident. Placebo effects and the effects of relief from vasomotor symptoms were not controlled for. However, in an earlier study, Sherwin and Gelfand (1985) did find positive effects of oestrogen upon mood in a placebo controlled cross-over trial. In another study, Myers, Dixen, Morrissette et al. (1990) included a placebo condition, and compared this with oestrogen regimens. Vasomotor symptoms reduced but no changes in mood were reported, as assessed by daily rating scales. In an attempt to overcome the confounding effects of vasomotor symptom relief, Ditkoff, Crary, Cristo and Lobo (1991) conducted a randomized double blind study of thirty six asymptomatic Hispanic American women, all of whom had undergone hysterectomy. Oestrogen (0.625), oestrogen (1.25) and a placebo condition were compared. There were small (2 scale points) but significant decreases in depressed mood, as assessed by the Beck Depression Scale, for both treated groups, but no dose response. However, all the women scored within the normal range in this study. Sherwin and Gelfand (1989) compared the same doses as Ditkoff, Crary, Cristo and Lobo, and, while there was no placebo condition, those taking the 1.25 dose reported significantly more elation, better sleep and greater well-being than those taking the 0.625 dose. The oestrogen levels of the 1.25 dose were considered by the authors to be in the supra-physiological range, suggesting that there may be a positive effect of oestrogen upon well-being when higher doses of oestrogen are used.

## Theoretical implications

Epidemiological studies do not support the claim that depressed mood or other psychological symptoms necessarily increase at the menopause, and certainly the cross-cultural variation in experience casts doubt upon the notion of an essentially biological cause of distress at this time. While it remains possible that hormonal changes might influence mood for some women, the effects of psychosocial factors are likely to be greater for the majority.

Further problems exist for the biomedical model since no clear correlation is evident between oestrogen levels and reports of depressive symptoms. In addition, there is no conclusive evidence that oestrogen therapy improves depressed mood in clinic samples, over and above placebo effects. (There is slightly more evidence of improvements in treated women who have previously undergone surgical menopause.) There is some evidence – but again it is equivocal – of a small improvement in well-being in selected healthy samples and there may be a dose response. However, even if it were conclusively proved to be the case, the reasons for treating healthy women or encouraging them to use a pharmacological agent to 'feel better' should obviously be questioned – particularly when the majority of women do not feel more depressed during the menopause, and the major causal factors of depressed mood appear to be psychosocial in nature.

In support of biological influences is the finding that chronic ill-health often precipitates chronic depression. Severe vasomotor symptoms, an early menopause and surgical menopause have also been found to be associated with depressed mood. In addition, psychosocial factors, such as life stress, might influence hormone levels.

Feminist writers have noted the ways in which scientific and medical views perpetuate sexism and ageism by reinforcing the idea that the menopause is a necessarily negative event and that the postmenopausal women is deficient, having to be treated for 'irritability, depression and loss of libido'. In other words, these women's problems are individualized and the social structures which maintain the relatively low status of older women in western societies are ignored (Greer, 1991; Hunter, 1990b; Worcester and Whatley, 1992).

Both biomedical and sociocultural models share a determinism which neglects women's differences and their own opinions about the menopause and its 'treatment'. At the same time purely psychological models can be criticized for blaming the woman for her emotional reactions during the menopause. The biomedical and the sociocultural discourses present polarized images of menopausal women – either at risk of developing numerous physical and emotional problems, or having no or few problems. Clearly, the full range of experiences of women are unlikely to be represented by either model.

The extent to which women themselves have been influenced by the medical model is uncertain. For example, in a recent North American study of women's attitudes, the majority felt that the menopause should be 'viewed as a medical condition and treated as such'. Although, at the same time, they attributed emotional problems to life events rather than hormonal changes, and preferred non-hormonal treatment options to HRT (Leiblum and Swartzman, 1986). Doctors, perhaps not surprisingly, tend to regard the menopause as more pathological than do women (Cowan, Warren and Young, 1985). Kaufert and Gilbert (1986), after reviewing the available evidence, concluded that in practice the menopause has not been medicalized to any great extent when compared to pregnancy and childbirth. In fact, uptake and adherence rates for HRT are generally thought to be low. Approximately 10 per cent of 45 to 55 year old women in Britain use the treatment, and of those starting HRT a considerable proportion discontinue within the first six months (Spector, 1989; Bryce and Lilford, 1990). In a qualitative study, Martin (1987) found that the vast majority of older women saw the menopause in a positive light; younger women tended to share the medical view of the menopause. She concluded that 'women choose – at least to some extent – whether or not to treat ... menopause as a medical event'. Future qualitative research could usefully explore the various meanings of the menopause and the discourses used by women themselves (Dickson, 1990).

A biopsychosocial model would seem to be the most appropriate framework within which to understand the above findings. In the biopsychosocial model, Figure 4.1, the woman's internal representation of the menopause is seen as central. The meaning of the menopause and the personal implications this has for a woman are understood in terms of her psychosocial and cultural context, as well as her experience of physical changes. This model is discussed in detail in Hunter (1994); clinical and practical implications are discussed in the next section.

From a socio-political perspective, changes that improve the opportunities and status of mid-aged and older women, for example help in caring for elderly relatives and appreciation of the economic value of experienced women, might

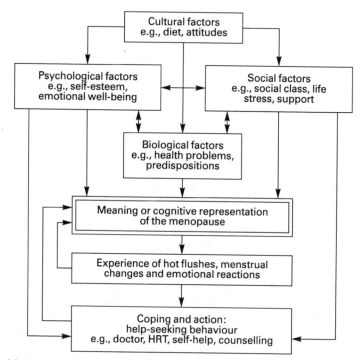

**Figure 4.1** A biopsychosocial model of the menopause

be expected to have general benefits to health and well-being, as well as to their experience of the menopause. Attempts to challenge the negative stereotyped beliefs which surround menopause and ageing, and which have adverse effects upon women's well-being, should be encouraged.

Women and doctors should be fully informed about the menopause and HRT with *balanced* information, based on the available evidence. If women (and their friends and families) are prepared – by being informed, having realistic beliefs, and a knowledge of a range of treatments and methods available to alleviate symptoms that might arise (Hunter, 1990b) – they are likely to approach the menopause with a sense of greater personal control and fewer fears. The effects of providing 45 year old women with information and discussion of beliefs, as well as health education, is currently being evaluated (Liao and Hunter, in preparation).

Women who do seek help during the menopause are not necessarily representative of menopausal women in general. They are likely to be experiencing more emotional and physical problems. If depression does occur at this time, a hormonal cause should not be automatically assumed. It is important to take time to enquire about the woman's individual views and circumstances. The following factors can be considered:

1. the psychological significance of the menopause, including mixed feelings about fertility and ageing,
2. reactions to social attitudes towards older women, for example feeling embarrassed or devalued,

3. anxiety and uncertainty about the process of the menopause transition, e.g. irregular periods, not knowing how long it might last,
4. reactions to vasomotor symptoms, which might affect sleep, and
5. coincidental life problems, chronic ill-health, marital problems and role changes.

Clarification of the problem is often all that is needed, using a biopsychosocial framework to discuss the possible influences and their interactions. For women who do feel depressed and want help, psychological therapies, such as cognitive behaviour therapy, can be used to help people to find appropriate solutions to their problems (Greene and Hart, 1987; Hunter, 1994). However, in practice, there is a dearth of alternative treatment choices for women. Problem-solving groups for women who feel stressed or depressed during midlife are currently being evaluated in general practice (Hunter and Liao, 1995a). Support groups are also used to share information, problems and remedies. Many women are interested in dietary modifications and exercise for well-being and general health. These measures are also recommended because adequate calcium together with weight-bearing exercise appears to help prevent the development of osteoporosis (Gannon, 1988). For women who have hot flushes but who do not want to have HRT, a cognitive-relaxation treatment has been developed (Hunter and Liao, 1995b). Provisional results suggest that this treatment might well be beneficial.

Finally, emotional reactions or mixed feelings resulting from a reappraisal of the past and thoughts about the future are obviously not abnormal. The menopause can provide a useful focus, a time for women to consider their own health and well-being, especially as, on average, one third of a woman's life is spent after the menopause.

## Further reading

Hunter, M. (1990). *Your Menopause*. London: Pandora Press.
Hunter, M. (1994). *Counselling in Obstetrics and Gynaecology*. Leicester: British Psychological Society.

## Applications

### 1. Prevention
Changes that improve the opportunities and status of mid-aged and older women might be expected to have general benefits to health and well-being as well as to their experience of the menopause. Challenges to the negative stereotypes which surround menopause and ageing should be encouraged.

### 2. Treatment
Women and doctors need to be fully informed about the menopause and HRT with balanced information, based on available evidence.

Depression which occurs during the menopause is not necessarily due to hormonal changes. The individual woman's views and life circumstances should be assessed, including: the psychological significance of menopause for her, her reactions to social attitudes towards older women, any concerns she has about the process of the menopausal transition (e.g. how long it will last, irregular periods), her reactions to vasomotor symptoms and any effects they might have on sleep patterns, other problems in her life, e.g. chronic ill-health, marital problems, role changes. For women who do feel depressed and want help, cognitive behaviour therapy may be useful, and other psychosocial interventions are currently being evaluated.

# References

Alder, E. M., Bancroft, J. and Livingstone, J. (1992). Estadiol implants, hormone levels and reported symptoms. *Psychosomatic Obstetrics and Gynaecology*, **13**, 223–35.

Asso, D. (1983). *The Real Menstrual Cycle*. Avon: Wiley and Son.

Avis, N. E. and McKinlay, S. M. (1991) A longitudinal analysis of women's attitudes towards the menopause: results from the Massachusetts Women's Health Study. *Maturitas*, **13**, 65–79.

Avis, N. E., Kaufert, P. A., McKinlay, S. A. and Vass, K. (1993). The evolution of menopausal symptoms. In *The Menopause* (H. G. Burger, ed.) London: Balliere Tindall.

Aylward, M. (1976). Oestrogens, plasma tryptophan levels in peri-menopausal patients. In *The Management of the Menopause and Post Menopausal Years* (S. Campbell, ed.) Baltimore: University Pak Press.

Ballinger, C. B. (1990). Psychiatric aspects of the menopause. *British Journal of Psychiatry*, **156**, 773–81.

74    Reproductive Potential and Fertility Control

Ballinger, C. B., Browning, M. C. K. and Smith, A. H. W. (1987). Hormone profiles and psychological symptoms in peri-menopausal women. *Maturitas*, **9**, 235–51.

Ballinger, S. (1985). Psychosocial stress and symptoms of menopause: a comparative study of menopause clinic patients and non-patients. *Maturitas*, **7**, 315–27.

Ballinger, S., Cobbin, D., Krivanek, J. and Saunders, D. (1979). Life stresses and depression in the menopause. *Maturitas*, **1**, 191–9.

Beyenne, Y. (1986). Cultural significance and physiological manifestations of menopause, a biocultural analysis. *Culture, Medicine and Psychiatry*, **10**, 47–71.

Boulet, M., Lehert, P. H. and Riphagen, F. E. (1985). The menopause viewed in relation to other life events – a study performed in Belgium. *Maturitas*, **10**, 333–42.

Brinton, L. A. (1990). Menopause and the risk of breast cancer. *Annals New York Academy of Sciences*, 357–62.

Brown, G. W. and Harris, T. (1978). *Social Origins of Depression*. London: Tavistock Publications.

Bryce, F. C. and Lilford, R. J. (1991). General practitioners use of hormone replacement therapy in Yorkshire. *European Journal of Obstetrics and Gynaecology*, **37**, 55–61.

Bungay, G. T., Vessay, M. P. and McPherson, C. K. (1980). Study of symptoms in middle life with special reference to the menopause. *British Medical Journal*, **ii**, 181–3.

Campbell, S. (1976). Double blind psychometric studies on the effects of natural oestrogens on postmenopausal women. In *The Management of the Menopause and Postmenopausal Years* (S. Campbell, ed.). Lancaster: MTP Press.

Cooke, D. J. and Greene, J. G. (1981). Types of life events in relation to symptoms at the climacterium. *Journal of Psychosomatic Research*, **25**, 5–11.

Coope, J. (1981). Is oestrogen therapy effective in the treatment of menopausal depression? *Journal of the Royal College of General Practitioners*, **31**, 134–40.

Cowan, G., Warren, L. W. and Young, J. L. (1985). Medical perceptions of menopausal symptoms. *Psychology of Women Quarterly*, **9**, 1, 3–14.

Dennerstein, L., Burrows, G. D., Hyman, C. and Sharpe, K. (1979). Hormone therapy and affect. *Maturitas*, **1**, 247–59.

Dickson, G. L. (1990). A feminist poststructural analysis of the knowledge of menopause. *Advances in Nursing Science*, **12**, 3, 15–31.

Ditkoff, E. C., Crary, W. G., Cristo, M. and Lobo, R. A. (1991). Estrogen improves psychological function in asymptomatic postmenopausal women. *Obstetrics and Gynaecology*, **78**, 6, 991–5.

Flint, M. (1975). The menopause: reward or punishment. *Psychosomatics*, **16**, 161–3.

Gannon, L. (1988). The potential role of exercise in the alleviation of menstrual disorders and menopausal symptoms: a theoretical synthesis of recent research. *Women and Health*, **14**, 2, 105–27.

Gath, D. and Iles, S. (1990). Depression and the menopause. *British Medical Journal*, **300**, 1287–8.

Gath, D., Osborn, M., Bungay, G., Iles, S., Day, A., Bond, A. and Passingham, C. (1987). Psychiatric disorder and gynaecological symptoms in middle aged women; a community survey. *British Medical Journal*, **294**, 213–18.

Glenn, N. D. (1975). Psychological well-being in the post parent stage: some evidence from national surveys. *Journal of Marriage and Family*, **37**, 105–10.

Greene, J. G. (1984). *The Social and Psychological Origins of the Climacteric Syndrome*. Aldershot: Gower.

Greene, J. G. and Cooke, D. J. (1980). Life stress and symptoms at the climacterium. *British Journal of Psychiatry*, **136**, 486–91.

Greene, J. G. and Hart, D. M. (1987). The evaluation of a psychological treatment programme for menopausal women. *Maturitas*, **9**, 1, 41–8.

Greer, G. (1991).*The Change*. London: Hamish Hamilton.

Hallstrom, T. (1973). *Mental Disorder and Sexuality in the Climacteric: A Study in Psychiatric Epidemiology*. Göteborg, Sweden: Scandinavian University Books.

Holte, A. (1992). Influences of natural menopause on health complaints; a prospective study of healthy Norwegian women. *Maturitas*, **14**, 2, 127–41.

Hunter, M. S. (1988). Psychological and somatic experience of the climacteric and postmenopause: predicting individual differences and helpseeking behaviour. University of London: unpublished PhD thesis.

Hunter, M. S. (1990a). Emotional well-being, sexual behaviour and hormone replacement therapy. *Maturitas*, **12**, 299–314.

Hunter, M. S. (1990b). *Your Menopause*. London: Pandora Press.

Hunter, M. S. (1992a). The S.E. England longitudinal study of the climacteric and postmenopause. *Maturitas*, **14**, 2, 117–26.

Hunter, M. S. (1992b). The Women's Health Questionnaire: a measure of physical and emotional well-being in mid-aged women. *Psychology and Health*, **7**, 45–54.

Hunter, M. S. (1994). *Counselling in Obstetrics and Gynaecology*. Leicester: British Psychological Society.

Hunter, M. S. and Liao, K. L. M. (1955a) Problem-solving groups for mid-aged women in general practice: a pilot study. *Journal of Reproductive and Infant Psychology*, (in press).

Hunter, M. S. and Liao, K. L. M. (1995b) Evaluation of a four-session cognitive-behavioural intervention for menopausal hot flushes. *British Journal of Health Psychology*, (in press).

Jaszmann, N. D. (1973). Epidemiology of the climacteric and postmenopause. In *Ageing and Oestrogens* (P. van Keep and C. Lauritzen, eds). Basel: Karger.

Jaszmann, N. D., van Lith, N. D. and Zaat, J. C. A. (1969). The peri-menopausal symptoms: the statistical analysis of a survey. *Medicine, Gynaecology and Sociology*, **4**, 10, 268–77.

Jennings, S., Mazaik, C. and McKinlay, S. (1984). Women and work: an investigation of the association between health and employment status in middle-aged women. *Social Science and Medicine*, **4**, 423–31.

Kaufert, P. (1982). Anthropology and the menopause: the development of a theoretical framework. *Maturitas*, **4**, 181–93.

Kaufert, P. A. (1984). Women and their health in the middle years: a Manitoba project. *Social Science and Medicine*, **18**, 3, 279–81.

Kaufert, P. A. and Gilbert, P. (1986). Women, menopause and medicalisation. *Culture Medicine and Psychiatry*, **10**, 7–21.

Kaufert, P. A. and Gilbert, P. (1988). Researching the symptoms of the menopause: an exercise in methodology. *Maturitas*, **10**, 2, 117–31.

Kaufert, P. A., Gilbert, P. and Tate, R. (1992). The Manitoba Project; a re-examination of the relationship between menopause and depression. *Maturitas*, **14**, 2, 143–56.

Klaiber, E. L., Broverman, D. M. and Vogel, W. (1972). The effects of oestrogen therapy on plasma MAO activity and EEG driving responses of depressed women. *American Journal of Psychiatry*, **128**, 1429–98.

Klaiber, E. L., Broverman, D. M., Vogel, W. and Korbayasti, V. (1979). Oestrogen therapy for severe persistent depression in women. *Archives of General Psychiatry*, **36**, 550–54.

Krafft-Ebbing, R. van (1877). Uber Imesin in Klimakterium. *Psychiatry*, **34**, 407.

Krystal, S. and Chiriboga, D. A. (1979). The empty nest process in mid-life men and women. *Maturitas*, **1**, 215–22.

Leiblum, S. R. and Swartzman, L. S. (1986). Women's attitudes about the menopause: an update. *Maturitas*, **81**, 47–56.

Lock, M. (1980). Ambiguities of aging: Japanese experience and perceptions of menopause. *Culture, Medicine and Psychiatry*, **10**, 23–46.

Martin, E. (1987). *The Woman in the Body*. Milton Keynes: Open University Press.

Matthews, K. A., Wing, R. R. and Kuller, L. H. (1990). Influences of natural menopause on psychological characteristics and symptoms of middle-aged healthy women. *J. Consult. Clin. Psychol.*, **58**, 345–63.

McCrea, F. B. (1983). The politics of the menopause: the discovery of a deficiency disease. *Social Problems*, **31**, 11–123.

McKinlay, S. M., Brambrilla, D. J. and Posner, J. (1992). The normal menopause transition. *Maturitas*, **14**, 2, 103–16.

McKinlay, S. M. and Jefferys, M. (1974). The menopausal syndrome. *British Journal of Preventative and Social Medicine*, **28**, 108–115.

McKinlay, M. and McKinlay, J. B. (1986). Health status and health care utilization by menopausal women. In *The Climacteric in Perspective* (M. Notelovitz and P. A. Van Keep, eds) Lancaster: MTP Press Ltd.

McKinlay, J. B., McKinlay, S. M. and Brambrilla, D. (1987). The relative contributions of endocrine changes and social circumstances to depression in mid-aged women. *Journal of Health and Social Behaviour*, **28**, 345–63.

Montgomery, J. C., Appelby, L., Brincat, M., Versi, E., Tapp, A., Fenwick, P. B. C. and Studd, J. W. W. (1987). Effect of oestrogen and testosterone implants on psychological disorders in the climacteric. *The Lancet*, Feb. 7, 297–9.

Myers, L. S., Dixen, D., Morrissette, M., Carmichael, M. and Davidson, J. M. (1990). Effects of estrogen, androgen and progestin on sexual psychophysiology and behaviour in postmenopausal women. *Journal of Clinical Endocrinology and Metabolism*, **70**, 4, 1124–31.

Neugarten, B. L. (1979). Time, age and the life-cycle. *American Journal of Psychiatry*, **136**, 887–94.

Neugarten, B. L, Wood, V., Kraines, R. J. and Loomis, B. (1963). Women's attitudes towards the menopause. *Vita Humana*, **6**, 140–51.

Oldenhave, A. (1991). *Well-being and Sexuality in the Climacteric*. Geneva: International Health Foundation.

Owen, E. J., Siddle, N. C., McGarrigle, H. T. and Pugh, M. A. (1992). 25 mg oestradial implants – the dosage of first choice for subcutaneous oestrogen replacement therapy. *British Journal of Obstetrics and Gynaecology*, **99**, 671–5.

Paganini-Hill, A., Ross, R. K. and Henderson, B. E. (1988). Postmenopausal oestrogen treatment and stroke: a prospective study. *British Medical Journal*, **297**, 519–22.

Payer, L. (1991). The menopause in various cultures. In *A Portrait of the Menopause* (H. Burger and M. Boulet, eds). Lancaster: Parthenon.

Richardson, S. (1993). The biological basis of the menopause. In *The Menopause* (H. Burger, ed.). London: Bailliere's Clinical Endocrinology and Metabolism.

Sherwin, B. B. (1988). Affective changes with estrogen and androgen replacement therapy in surgically menopausal women. *Journal of Affective Disorders*, **14**, 177–87.

Sherwin, B. B. and Gelfand, M. M. (1985). Sex steroids and affect in the surgical menopause: a double-blind cross-over study. *Psychoneuroendocrinology*, **10**, 325–35.

Sherwin, B. B. and Gelfand, M. M. (1989). A prospective one-year study of estrogen and progestin in postmenopausal women: effects on clinical symptoms and lipoprotein lipids. *Obstetrics and Gynaecology*, **73**, 5, 759–66.

Smith, R. (1990). *Osteoporosis 1990*. London: Royal College of Physicians.

Spector, T. D. (1989). Use of oestrogen replacement therapy in high risk groups in the United Kingdom. *British Medical Journal*, **299**, 1434–5.

Studd, J. W. W. and Smith, R. N. J. (1993). Oestradiol and testosterone implants in menopause. In *The Menopause* (H. Burger, ed.). London: Bailliere's Clinical Endocrinology and Metabolism.

Swartzman, L. C., Edelberg, R. and Kemmann, E. (1990). Impact of stress on objectively recorded menopausal hot flushes and on flush report bias. *Health Psychology*, **9**, 529–45.

Thompson, B., Hart, S. A. and Durno, D. (1973). Menopausal age and symptomatology in a general practice. *Journal of Biosocial Science*, **5**, 71–82.

Thompson, J. and Oswald, I. (1977). Effect of oestrogen on the sleep, mood and anxiety of menopausal women. *British Medical Journal*, **2**, 1317–19.

Ussher, J. M. (1992). Research and theory into human reproduction. *British Journal of Clinical Psychology*, **31**, 129–51.

Utian, W. H. (1975). Definitive symptoms of post-menopause incorporating use of vaginal parabasal cell index. In *Frontiers in Hormone Research: Oestrogens in the Post-Menopause* (P. A. van Keep and C. Lauritzen, eds). Basel: Karger.

Utian, W. (1977). Current status of menopause and postmenopausal estrogen therapy. In *Obstetrics and Gynaecology Survey*. Baltimore: Williams and Wilkins.

Walfisch, S. Antonovsky, H. and Maoz, B. (1984). Relationship between biological changes, symptoms and health behaviour during the climacteric. *Maturitas*, **6**, 9–17.

Wilbush, J. (1979). La menespausie – the birth of a syndrome, *Maturitas*, **1**, 145–51.

Wilbush, J. (1984). Clinical information – signs, semeions and symptoms: discussion paper. *Journal of the Royal Society of Medicine*, **77**, 766–73.

Wilson, R. A. (1966). *Feminine Forever*. New York: Evans.

Worcester, N. and Whatley, M. H. (1992). The selling of HRT: Playing the fear factor. *Feminist Review*, **41**.

World Health Organisation (1981). *Research on the Menopause*. Geneva: WHO.

# 5

# Psychological aspects of gynaecological procedures

**Pauline Rafferty and Susan Williams**

The first four chapters were concerned with psychosocial aspects of normal reproductive potential. The explanation of processes like menstruation and menopause in terms of illness or disease, and their subsequent medicalization, has been shown to be a very limited way of understanding normal physiological processes. There are times, though, when medical intervention is appropriate, in preventing or treating conditions specific to the reproductive organs. In this chapter Pauline Rafferty and Susan Williams consider the psychosocial aspects of the procedures which women may experience either in order to detect abnormalities at an early stage or to treat them. They focus particularly on examinations of the cervix through 'smear' tests or colposcopy and on the surgical removal of the uterus, hysterectomy. How do women feel about internal examinations? Does a hysterectomy cause depression or make women less 'feminine'? How do women cope with gynaecological procedures?

## Introduction

Gynaecological procedures can be defined as any procedure used to screen for or investigate and treat abnormality or disease of the female reproductive organs (see Figure 5.1). Their associations with fertility and malignancy are recognized as being extremely stressful to women (Wallace, 1984). Before a woman undergoes a gynaecological procedure, she may have been through various stages in

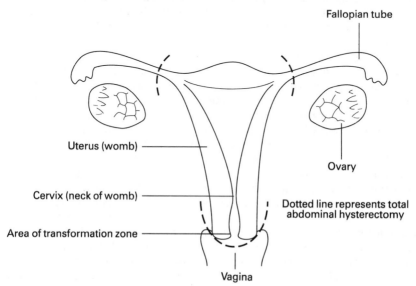

**Figure 5.1** Front view of female reproduction organs

the health care system. Often, women consult their GP with symptoms such as pelvic pain or abnormal bleeding. Sometimes, abnormalities are identified in asymptomatic women through screening in GP surgeries or well-woman and family planning clinics. For example a woman may have an abnormal cervical smear or an examination may reveal a fibroid in her uterus. For certain symptoms, the GP may initially treat the woman, for example, by prescribing drugs to control pelvic pain or abnormal bleeding. These treatments may be unsuccessful or may require surgical intervention and therefore the woman may be referred for an outpatient appointment with a gynaecologist. At this stage, the woman may have a further internal examination or the consultation may consist of a discussion of her symptoms only. The gynaecologist may feel an investigative procedure such as laparoscopy or D and C is necessary or may perform a minor procedure to treat, for example, an abnormal smear using colposcopy or to cauterize genital warts. Women with certain conditions may require major gynaecological surgery such as hysterectomy. Descriptions of some of the more common procedures which illustrate the variety and range of treatments and care, in their different settings, are outlined below.

## Types of gynaecological procedures

### Cervical screening

Cervical screening refers to the taking and subsequent laboratory examination of endocervical cells from the transformation zone (Figure 5.1) of the cervix. Screening is offered to all sexually active women between the ages of 20 and 60 years in Scotland (25 to 64 years in England, Wales and Northern Ireland). The transformation zone is an area of change and high cell activity where the nuclei of cells may show abnormal characteristics which are known to be a precursor to cancer of the cervix. Any woman who has had heterosexual sex is at risk of having an abnormal smear and screening is designed to identify abnormalities of the cervix before cancer develops. In some areas of Britain one in twenty smears is abnormal (McIlwaine 1994, personal communication). Screening commonly takes place at GPs' surgeries and to a lesser extent at well-woman and family planning clinics. The introduction of the GP contract with payment for reaching target levels for cervical screening (Department of Health, 1990) has meant that family doctors are paid more if women are screened at their surgeries. Population screening through call and recall systems is now in operation, replacing the somewhat opportunistic basis by which women were previously screened. This was disliked by many women who felt distressed and embarrassed when asked to undergo an unexpected intimate examination during a visit to their GP for a different reason (Williams, 1992).

Cervical screening although not associated with pain is regarded as embarrassing and undignified by most women. The taking of a smear involves the woman lying on her back with legs apart and the insertion of a speculum to keep the vagina open. The cervix is then visualized before exfoliated cells of the transformation zone are collected using a special spatula or brush. The cells are quickly transferred to a slide and placed in a fixative before being sent to a cytology laboratory for close examination using a microscope. The significance of any abnormality, for individual women, cannot be determined at this stage. Slightly abnormal smears (mild dyskaryosis) often regress without treatment and just require more frequent smears to ensure this has happened. Even more severe abnormalities (moderate or severe dyskaryosis) may have no significance, but, for some women, the abnormalities need to be investigated and if necessary treated with colposcopy since they indicate that cancer may develop in the future.

## Colposcopy

Colposcopy is an outpatient procedure mainly used for diagnosis and treatment of abnormal cervical smears. It involves a microscopic look at the cervix using a colposcope which looks like a large pair of binoculars on a stand. The colposcope does not go inside the body. It does not require anaesthetic and in clinical, medical terms this is a minor procedure, similar to that for taking a cervical smear. After visualizing and examining the cervix, the doctor identifies areas of abnormality and takes a biopsy which leads to a much more accurate diagnosis than the smear. In some clinics treatment takes place immediately after the biopsy is taken. In others a return outpatient appointment is made and treatment takes place according to the biopsy diagnosis.

There are several methods of treatment all of which totally destroy the abnormal cells (Anderson, Jordan, Morse and Sharp, 1992). Outpatient treatment is medically easy and does not require a general anaesthetic. If the area of abnormality extends up the cervical canal and cannot be totally visualized it is necessary for the woman to be admitted to hospital for surgical removal (cone biopsy) of the affected tissue under general anaesthetic. All types of treatment for abnormal cervical cells are virtually 100 per cent successful (Centre for Disease Control, 1990) and it is unusual for abnormal cells to recur.

## Other investigative and diagnostic procedures

Some of the most common procedures are those used to diagnose and investigate gynaecological problems such as acute or chronic pain, abnormal bleeding and infertility. Laparoscopy is the direct inspection of the ovaries, fallopian tubes and contents of the uterus (Gould, 1990). This procedure is also used for sterilization. It is carried out under general anaesthetic using a laparoscope inserted through the abdominal wall. Length of stay in hospital depends on the reason for the laparoscopy but overnight stay is usually required. Although a minor procedure, it can be stressful to women because of what it may indicate about malignancy or fertility.

Hysterosalpingography is a diagnostic X-ray examination of the genital tract and is used as a test for patency of the fallopian tubes and to detect abnormality of the uterus. Normally, it is carried out during menstruation so as not to disturb an undiagnosed pregnancy. Radio-opaque dye is inserted into the genital tract via the cervix and the progress of the dye is observed on a television screen. If the tubes are open dye leaks into the pelvic cavity. Some pain may be experienced at this stage which may require analgesia. The procedure is usually carried out, without anaesthetic, in an outpatient department or in a day care unit.

Dilatation and curettage (D and C) refers to the widening of the cervical canal and the scraping away of the lining of the uterus. Hysteroscopy is the microscopic examination of the inside of the uterus undertaken at the same time as D and C. The procedure requires a general anaesthetic and is commonly carried out in a day care unit. Hysteroscopy with D and C can be used as a diagnostic procedure to identify abnormalities of the uterus, the cause of abnormal or post-menopausal bleeding and to establish if ovulation has occurred.

## Major gynaecological procedures

**Hysterectomy**, the most common major gynaecological procedure, is the overall term used for removal of the uterus (see Figure 5.1). Sometimes secondary organs such as ovaries and fallopian tubes are removed at the same time (Barnes and Chamberlain, 1988). Hysterectomy is generally viewed by gynaecologists as a clinically major event. In Britain admission to hospital is required and a general anaesthetic is usually given. The operation can be carried out via an incision through the abdomen or via the vagina which leaves no visible scar. Post-operative recovery usually involves about eight days in hospital and around six weeks convalescing at home (Evans and Richardson, 1988). Full recovery is recognized to take several weeks and women are commonly advised to take three months off work.

Hysterectomy is performed for a variety of reasons including long-term menstrual bleeding abnormalities such as menorrhagia (heavy bleeding) and inter-menstrual bleeding; endometriosis; fibroids; cancer of the uterus or cervix; pelvic inflammatory disease; abdominal pain; dysmenorrhea (pain during menstruation); and prolapse of the uterus and/or vagina (Barnes and Chamberlain, 1988). Some of these indications are symptoms (such as menorrhagia and dysmenorrhea) and others are diagnoses or causes of symptoms (such as cancer of the uterus). Hysterectomy is often recommended when other forms of treatment fail (Rees, 1981). For example, menorrhagia and dysmenorrhea can be treated using various endocrine or non-steroidal anti-inflammatory drugs.

**Endometrial ablation** is a recently developed, more minor procedure which may be used instead of hysterectomy. It is most commonly undertaken for menorrhagia when a hysterectomy is unsuitable or unwanted. The procedure involves the examination and destruction of the lining of the uterus (endometrium) using a laser beam. Drugs are given to prepare the endometrium and to stop menstruation for at least six weeks before ablation. The procedure requires a general anaesthetic but is commonly carried out in a hospital day care unit. Ablation stops or greatly reduces menstruation. However, if only a small part of the endometrium remains, pregnancy can occur. Endometrial ablation can be particularly useful for women suffering from physical disability (e.g. multiple sclerosis) who find coping with menstruation difficult. In these cases, the gynaecological procedure is used to improve a woman's life when no gynaeco-logical abnormality occurs.

**Pelvic floor repair** is used to treat prolapse of the uterus. This is 'the descent of the uterus into, or through the vagina or the ... "bulging" of the structures adjacent to the vagina, into the vagina' (Farrer, 1985). Surgical repair may be chosen in preference to use of a ring pessary or hysterectomy. Prolapse occurs most often in menopausal women who have had children and prevention involves good midwifery and obstetric care. Conditions which increase abdomimal pressure (e.g. obesity, tumours and chronic constipation) can also exacerbate the problem. It is a particularly stressful condition to women because besides backache and a dragging pain in the vagina, there is also the association with urinary incontinence if the bladder is displaced by the sagging uterus. Vaginal repair of a utero-vaginal prolapse (colporrhaphy) aims to restore strength and support to the vaginal walls. Success of vaginal repair operations is not well documented. It has been estimated that in up to 20 per cent of cases the problem recurs (Fergusson, 1984).

## Psychosocial aspects of gynaecological procedures

The psychological impact on a woman of a gynaecological procedure may bear little relationship to medical assessment of importance. Even a vaginal examination, considered medically quite trivial, may be a fairly major event in a woman's life. During this procedure the woman's genitals are examined and may be palpated and the doctor often inserts a speculum to examine the cervix and vagina. Women often have negative attitudes towards this examination and have reported feelings of degradation and fear (Areskog-Wijma, 1987). A male gynaecologist is perceived as making the experience more traumatic and many women, when asked, say they would prefer a female doctor (Areskog-Wijma, 1987; Ivins and Kent, 1993). These women felt that a woman would be better able to provide sympathy and understanding during examinations. A Swedish study reported that women with such preferences were significantly more likely to report feelings of degradation associated with the examination (Areskog-Wijma, 1987).

Wijma and Areskog-Wijma (1987) have pointed out the different 'frames of reference' which the gynaecologist and the woman have about gynaecological examinations. The doctor has a medical framework which makes the consultation 'safe and filled with routines'. Doctors imply that women should also take this point of view (Emerson, 1970). Women, however, take a different view when they have to show their genitals, their most intimate parts, to a stranger. Society has set up taboos and even laws against the showing of genitals and during gynaecological examinations these must be broken. Showing and touching of the genitals has sexual associations and is usually done in the context of mutual trust and closeness (Settlage, 1975). A woman may be uncomfortable, therefore, with having someone look at and touch her genitals outside this context.

Gynaecological procedures are associated with high levels of anxiety (Johnston, 1980; Wallace, 1983) and some women experience very severe distress which may last for some time. The Spielberger State-Trait Anxiety Inventory (STAI) has been used with patients undergoing gynaecological procedures (Spielberger, Gorsuch, Lushene et al., 1983). The STAI State scale is a twenty item scale which gives scores ranging from 20 to 80. The mean normative STAI State score for adult women is 35.2. STAI State scores of around 50 have been reported before colposcopy (Marteau, 1990; Wilkinson, Jones and McBride, 1990; Williams, 1992) and scores of around 40 have been reported for women awaiting gynaecological surgery (Johnston, 1980, 1987; Warrington and Gottlieb, 1987). While anxiety decreases post-operatively this decrease may not occur until around six days after surgery when women feel sure there have been no complications (Johnston, 1980).

Menage (1993) has reported cases of post-traumatic stress disorder (PTSD) following a variety of gynaecological and/or obstetric procedures in a sample of women recruited from press advertisements. Thirty women of the sample of 500 fulfilled the criteria for diagnosis of PTSD. These women were found to differ significantly from women who rated the experience as 'very good' to 'slightly distressing' in, for example, feelings of powerlessness during the procedure, lack of information, the experience of pain and a perceived lack of consent to the procedure.

# Wider issues surrounding gynaecological procedures

Colposcopy and hysterectomy by their diversity can be considered to be representative of gynaecological procedures both in terms of medical impact and women's experiences and responses. This section will, therefore, focus on issues associated with these two procedures.

### Issues associated with cervical screening and colposcopy

The success of treatment for abnormal cervical smears means that anxiety about outcome is nearly always groundless. The physiological and medical importance of having an abnormal cervical smear and its consequent treatment are however at variance with women's perceptions of the problem (Quilliam, 1989). Cervical screening is viewed by health professionals as a method for control of cervical cancer whereas women are more likely to view it as an opportunity to receive reassurance that they do not have cancer (McKie, 1993). Therefore, an abnormal smear result is contrary to many women's expectations. Both the perceived consequences of the result and anticipation of the colposcopy and treatment can cause substantial anxiety (Marteau, 1990; Wilkinson, Jones and McBride, 1990; Williams, 1992).

Screening and treatment of cervical abnormality have developed to prevent cervical cancer, however attention has only recently been paid to reducing the anxiety which many women experience. Most commonly this attention has focused on the information and support needs of women (Posner and Vesey, 1988; Quilliam, 1989; Barsevick and Lauverd, 1990; Wilkinson, Jones and McBride, 1990; Williams, 1992). These studies indicate that most women do not know the purpose of screening and the meaning and implications of an abnormal smear. They may be anxious and worried that they have cancer. For some women and their partners there is an association with promiscuity and some women describe themselves as 'feeling dirty' (Quilliam, 1989). Sexual relationships often suffer (Campion, Atia, Edwards et al., 1988). Women also have little knowledge of and are anxious about undergoing treatment and its success (Marteau, 1990; Barsevick and Lauverd, 1990). They may also be concerned about its effects on future childbearing.

In a study of 149 Canadian women, Nugent and Tamlyn-Leaman (1992) concluded that although seeking information is the most common coping mechanism in women following an abnormal smear, it is premature to provide information before determining what women already know and what they would like to know. They found that, amongst other things, women lack basic knowledge about location of the cervix and the meaning of an abnormal smear result and most (85 per cent) had no clear understanding of the relationship between an abnormal result and disease of the cervix. Only 27 per cent of women had a good understanding of the purpose of colposcopy. The findings are similar for Scottish women. As part of a multi-stage study, the knowledge status of 273 women was determined before the design of an information and support package (Williams, 1992). It was found that 31 per cent of the women knew the purpose of having a smear, only 4 per cent had an accurate picture of what was likely to be wrong (9 per cent thought they had cancer) and 43 per cent did not know what was involved at the colposcopy examination (23 per cent had some in-depth knowledge). Interestingly, there was no significant association between knowledge status and perceived levels of coping or anxiety in this study.

Not all women, however, want in-depth information. It has been shown that individuals differ in their style of coping with threatening situations, including medical procedures (Miller, 1980). Miller (1980) has proposed that coping style should be assessed in terms of monitoring and blunting. She suggests that individuals tend to cope with stressful situations by gathering information related to the threat ('monitors') or by using distraction ('blunters'). Studies have examined how coping style affects the process of coping and the outcome of coping attempts. Those classified as 'monitors' have been found to want more information about the forthcoming medical procedure (Miller and Mangan, 1983; Steptoe and O'Sullivan, 1986). In a study of colposcopy patients, Miller and Mangan (1983) found that 'monitors' were significantly more dissatisfied with the information they had received than were 'blunters'. Similarly, Steptoe and O'Sullivan (1986) reported that 'monitors' wanted more information than 'blunters' about their forthcoming gynaecological surgery. 'Monitors' in this study also had more knowledge about the surgical procedures (Steptoe and O'Sullivan, 1986). Despite the increased knowledge of 'monitors', 'blunters' have been found to have a better adjustment to medical procedures and have been found to be less anxious during the procedure (Miller, 1988). This is thought to be because 'blunters' are better at distracting themselves from the more threatening aspects of the procedure.

Coping style has also been found to interact with the amount of information women are given before a stressful medical procedure. Miller and Mangan (1983) gave their sample of colposcopy patients either voluminous preparatory information or minimal information about the procedure. Immediately before the procedure, the only group to show a significant decrease in pulse rate were the 'blunters' who had received a low level of information. At the end of the procedure, 'monitors' who had been given a large amount of information had lowered pulse rates but the pulse rate remained high in 'monitors' given little information and 'blunters' given voluminous information, an interaction which was statistically significant.

These findings have been used to suggest that patients' coping styles should be established in order to determine whether and what type of preparation they require for the medical procedure (Mathews and Ridgeway, 1984; Miller, 1988). However, the general screening of patients is likely to prove impractical in clinical settings and no reports have been made of this practice. A different approach is being implemented by Williams (1994). Procedural, sensory, coping and reassuring information is made available in a variety of forms (basic letter, booklets, video and audio tape) and in various stages. This is presented to women as a 'take as much as you want, how you want' approach to information giving and is a practical attempt to tailor preparation to individual coping style.

## Issues associated with hysterectomy

In the nineteenth and early twentieth centuries, most women's illnesses were believed to be caused by disorder of the uterus. The uterus was seen as the dominant female organ and it was believed to be connected to every other organ in the female body (Hufnagel, 1988). Hysterectomy became common practice by 1890 as the only method of relieving gonorrhea which was rife at that time (Hufnagel, 1988).

Early writers discussed the loss of the uterus in terms of a loss of female identity and concluded that women suffered depression and sexual problems as a result of this loss (e.g. Deutsch, 1945; Patterson and Craig, 1963). Early studies found high levels of psychiatric disorder following hysterectomy (Barker, 1968; Raphael, 1972; Richards, 1973, 1974). However these studies failed to assess levels of disorder before surgery. More recent studies have shown that psychiatric disorder is high before hysterectomy and is no higher or decreases after surgery (Moore and Tolley, 1976; Gath, Cooper and Day, 1982; Ryan, Dennerstein and Pepperell, 1989). These findings are in line with those which have found high levels of psychiatric disorder among gynaecology outpatients (Greenberg, 1983; Slade, Anderton and Faragher, 1988). Similarly, studies have shown that hysterectomy does not have a detrimental effect on women's sexuality after surgery (Wijma, 1984).

## Unnecessary surgery?

The belief that the uterus was the central female organ gave way to the idea that the only function of the uterus is for reproduction and therefore it should be removed when a woman's reproductive potential has ended. The 'useless uterus syndrome' has been described as a valid indication for hysterectomy (Sloan, 1978). In 1969 Wright, an American physician, wrote:

> The uterus has but one function: reproduction. After the last planned pregnancy, the uterus becomes a useless, bleeding, symptom producing, potentially cancer-bearing organ and therefore should be removed. If in addition both ovaries are removed ... another common source of inoperable malignancy is eliminated.

Since hysterectomy is a major surgical procedure which induces anxiety (Johnston, 1980) and is associated with several post-operative problems, it seems highly inappropriate and irresponsible to advocate the performance of the operation as a matter of course (Hufnagel, 1988; Travis, 1985). Travis (1985) has carried out cost-benefit analyses of hysterectomies carried out in the USA in terms of mortality, life expectancy, morbidity, psychological outcome, quality of life, and dollar expenditure. This revealed that hysterectomy was associated with high costs and relatively limited benefits. Travis (1985) suggests that the discrepancy in terms of decisions to perform hysterectomies when the benefits may be limited in individual cases may be due to, for example, sexism and the desire to prevent cancer occurring. Doctors in this country have been criticized for their failure to use conservative drug treatments for women with menstrual problems and their reliance on hysterectomy as a method to remove these problems (Rees, 1981).

## Preparation for medical procedures

Women with gynaecological problems may experience a power imbalance in that the health professionals have more knowledge than the patient about her condition and about possible investigations and treatments. It is difficult, therefore, for a woman to participate fully in decisions concerning her care. She may feel that 'the doctor knows best'. It is important for women to feel that they have consented fully to gynaecological procedures because, as described above, perceived lack of consent and lack of information about the procedures can lead to severe psychological distress after gynaecological procedures (Menage, 1993). Hufnagel (1988), writing about the USA, has stated that:

> The creation of informed consent laws, to teach women about the consequences of hysterectomy is important. These should include information about: what is hysterectomy; how is it performed; what are the possible complications.

Information giving may, therefore, give some of the power to women and enable them to make decisions about their care. Wallace (1983) has also pointed to the importance of information giving for informed consent before gynaecological procedures but has shown that information also reduces anxiety and improves recovery from surgery. This is in line with other studies which show the benefits of psychological preparation for gynaecological surgery.

Reviews of the efficacy of psychological preparation for surgery have concluded that prepared patients have a better outcome than those who receive a placebo intervention or standard care (Mumford, Schlesinger and Glass, 1982; Devine and Cook, 1983, 1986; Mathews and Ridgeway, 1984; Wallace, 1984; Hathaway, 1986; Weinman and Johnston, 1988).

Preparation for surgery, including gynaecological surgery, has included other types of psychological methods as well as information giving. The main types of psychological intervention used to prepare patients for surgery are described in Table 5.1. They are: information; behavioural instructions; relaxation; modelling; and cognitive coping training (Mathews and Ridgeway, 1984).

## Efficacy of preparation

Reviewers have discussed the relative efficacy of these different types of psychological preparation. Reviews which have discussed cognitive coping suggest that this type of intervention is particularly effective (Mathews and Ridgeway, 1984; Wallace, 1984; Ludwick-Rosenthal and Neufeld, 1988). Similarly, behavioural instruction is also considered to be effective as is relaxation training (Mathews and Ridgeway, 1984). Few reviews have suggested that reassurance alone is an effective intervention (Alberts, Lyons, Moretti and Erickson, 1989).

**Table 5.1** Types of psychological intervention

• **Information**
*Procedural information* involves a factual description about what will happen before, during and after surgery (e.g. Janis, 1958).
   *Sensory information* describes the sensations (sights, sounds, smells, feelings etc.) a patient can expect to experience during and after a medical procedure (Johnson et al., 1978; Reading, 1982).

• **Behavioural instructions**
This involves teaching patients skills which are considered beneficial when performed after surgery, for example deep breathing, coughing, turning in bed and leg and foot exercises (Lindemann and Van Aernam, 1971).

• **Relaxation**
*Behavioural relaxation techniques*, for example telling patients to 'let the lower jaw drop' and to 'keep the tongue quiet and resting' and to 'let the lips get soft' and telling patients to breathe slowly and rhymically (Flaherty and Fitzpatrick, 1978).
   *Hypnotic relaxation technique* involves simple, usually taped hypnotic instructions (e.g. Hart, 1980).

• **Cognitive coping training**
Cognitive coping involves instructing patients to change their thoughts about hospital and surgery to more realistic or positive ones. For example, Ridgeway and Mathews (1982) used a technique which instructs patients to work out what is worrying them, then to think of more positive thoughts with which to replace these worries and finally, to think more about the positive thoughts.

• **Modelling**
This is learning by watching others perform (Brannon and Feist, 1992). Usually, a film of an actor undergoing the procedure is viewed. The actor is seen to be overcoming anxiety and coping well with the procedure (Melamed, 1984; Ludwick-Rosenthal and Neufeld, 1988).

Reviews which have included comparable categories of intervention have concluded that the efficacy of information has been established (Mathews and Ridgeway, 1984; Wallace, 1984) and it has been suggested that sensory information in particular is effective (Mathews and Ridgeway, 1984). However a more systematic review of psychological intervention (Weinman and Johnston, 1988) concluded that while information alone was effective in reducing the number of drugs patients received and reducing their length of post-operative stay, it was not effective in improving other indices of recovery (such as pain and mood). Further, a meta-analysis (a systematic, statistical method of integrating research findings) by Mumford, Schlesinger and Glass (1982) concluded that 'psychotherapeutic' interventions (i.e. reassurance, relaxation, and one study of cognitive coping) were associated with a larger effect than educational interventions (i.e. information). A combination of both types of intervention resulted in the largest effect.

In her study on the development and evaluation of preparatory information for women undergoing minor gynaecological surgery, Wallace found that, if asked to choose, procedural information was judged to be the most important but the preferred form of information is a combination of procedural, sensory, coping and reassuring information (Wallace, 1983). Therefore since most patients have been found to desire information before surgery and because patients require information for informed consent (Wallace, 1986), information giving as an intervention is justified and could lead to improved recovery if accompanied by other, 'psychological' elements.

## Summary and conclusions

This chapter has described several types of gynaecological procedures and has outlined the psychological implications of these procedures. It is important that the psychological aspects of gynaecological procedures are considered for the following reasons:

1. There is a high level of psychological disorder among gynaecological surgery patients (Greenberg, 1983; Slade, Anderton and Faragher, 1988). It has been suggested that some women who present with gynaecological problems have a psychiatric disorder which may make them more disturbed by their physical problems (Oates and Gath, 1989). Health professionals need to be able to identify those women whose reason for seeking medical help is influenced by their psychological state so that they do not recommend unnecessary gynaecological procedures.

2. The internal gynaecological examination and other gynaecological procedures are stressful to women (Johnston, 1980; Areskog-Wijma, 1987; Marteau, 1990; Menage, 1993). Psychological research has been involved in identifying factors, such as having a male gynaecologist, a perceived lack of control and lack of informed consent to the procedure which make the procedures particularly stressful. Health professionals can use this information to modify their encounters with gynaecology patients to reduce the stressful impact of the procedures. For example, they can ensure information is given to women about the procedure to facilitate informed consent.

   Psychological knowledge can also be used to train health professionals in the skills required to improve their interactions with gynaecology patients. For example, health professionals can learn listening skills, good use of questioning and learn to approach women with sensitivity and empathy (Hunter, 1994).

3. Psychologists have been involved in identifying women's need for information and in the design of psychological preparation for gynaecological procedures. The research has gone some way towards finding out which elements of the intervention are most successful and it has been suggested above that a combination of information and psychological elements (such as cognitive coping and relaxation training) is the most effective form of intervention. Psychological intervention is important for facilitating informed consent, empowering women and for improving women's adjustment to gynaecological procedures (i.e. reducing anxiety and improving recovery).

   Psychological research has also identified individual differences in styles of coping with stressful events including gynaecological procedures and this has lead to suggestions that psychological intervention should be tailored to suit coping style (Mathews and Ridgeway, 1984; Miller, 1988). A more practical approach has been suggested above which allows women to have as much information as they want in the form they want (Williams, 1992).

## Future directions for research

Most current research in this area has concentrated on the patients and the findings have implications for the service provided by health professionals.

Research is needed which focuses on those variables in the health professional–patient interaction which facilitate the gynaecological encounter and reduce the negative impact of the procedures. For example, do women prefer health professionals with a warm, empathetic manner or those with a more detached and professional approach? What aspects of the interaction make women feel they have no control over the procedure or have not fully consented to the procedure, i.e. what are the differences among women which make them more or less likely to experience extreme distress during a gynaecological procedure and what aspects of the gynaecological environment make this likely? This approach to the study of gynaecological procedures recognizes the range of individual differences among women in, for example, desire for information, as well as the differences of approach and skills which health professionals have and the complex interaction between the two.

## Applications

### Remember background
Women who undergo gynaecological procedures have often experienced distressing and debilitating symptoms for some time before referral to a gynaecologist. Alternatively a woman may have no symptoms and any abnormality diagnosed by screening may leave her totally unprepared.

### Reactions to the procedure
Many women, in addition to worry over the cause of symptoms or the result of screening tests, find gynaecological procedures very embarrassing. This may be especially so if the doctor is male.

### Anxiety
Gynaecological procedures are associated with high levels of anxiety which may last for some time. Information can reduce anxiety.

### Information needs
Coping style varies. Not all women want copious information and some cope better with none at all. Individual need should be addressed. Some women would prefer to see a video or listen to an audio tape in addition to, or in place of, written information. Content of information is important. Psychological preparation has been shown to reduce anxiety. Women also want sensory and reassuring information as well as that concerning facts.

# Further reading

Broome, A., Wallace, L. M. (eds) (1984). *Psychology and Gynaecological Problems*. New York: Tavistock.

Oates, M., Gath, D. (1989). Psychological aspects of gynaecological surgery. *Balliere's Clinical Obstetrics and Gynaecology*, **3**, 729–49.

Slade, P., Anderton, K. and Faragher, E. B. (1988). Psychological aspects of Gynaecological Outpatients. *Journal of Psychosomatic Obstetrics and Gynaecology*, **8**, 77–94.

# Referfences

Alberts, M. S., Lyons, J. S., Moretti, R. J. and Erickson, J. C. (1989). Psychological intervention in the pre-surgical period. *International Journal of Psychiatry in Medicine*, **19**, 91–106.

Anderson, M., Jordan, J., Morse, A. and Sharp, F. (1992). *A Text and Atlas of Integrated Colposcopy*. London: Chapman and Hall.

Areskog-Wijma, B. (1987). The gynaecological examination – women's experiences and preferences and the role of the gynaecologist. *Journal of Psychosomatic Obstetrics and Gynaecology*, **6**, 59–69.

Barker, M. G. (1968). Psychiatric illness after hysterectomy. *British Medical Journal*, ii, 91–5.

Barnes, J. and Chamberlain, G. (1988). *Lecture Notes on Gynaecology*. 2nd edn, London: Blackwell Scientific Publications.

Barsevick, A. and Lauverd, D. (1990). Women's information needs about colposcopy. *Journal of Nursing Scholarship*, **22**, 23–6.

Brannon, L. and Feist, J. (1992). *Health Psychology*. 2nd edn, Belmont, CA: Wadsworth Publishing.

Campion, M., Atia, W., Edwards, R., Cuzick, J. and Singer, A. (1988). Psychosexual trauma of an abnormal cervical smear. *British Journal of Obstetrics and Gynaecology*, **95**, 175–81.

Centre for Disease Control (1990). *Morbidity and Mortality Weekly Report*, **39**, 15, 246.

Deutsch, H. (1945). *The Psychology of Women*. New York: Grune and Stratton.

Devine, E. C. and Cook, T. D. (1983). A meta-analytic analysis of effects of psychoeducational intervention on length of postsurgical hospital stay. *Nursing Research*, **32**, 267–74.

Devine, E. C. and Cook, T. D. (1986). Clinical and cost-saving effects of psychoeducational intervention with surgical patients: a meta-analysis. *Research in Nursing and Health*, **9**, 89–105.

Emerson, J. (1970). Behaviour in private places. In *Recent Sociology*, No. 2 (P. Dreitzel, ed.). London: Macmillan.

Evans, C. and Richardson, P. H. (1988). Improved recovery and reduced post-operative stay after therapeutic suggestion during general anaesthesia. *Lancet*, Aug, 491–3.

Farrer, H. (1985). *Gynaecological Care*. 2nd edn, Melbourne: Pitman.

Fergusson, I. L. C. (1984). Genital prolapse. In *Contemporary Gynaecology* (G. Chamberlain, ed.) London: Butterworths.

Flaherty, G. G. and Fitzpatrick, J. J. (1978). Relaxation techniques to increase comfort level of postoperative patients: a preliminary study. *Nursing Research*, **27**, 352–5.

Gath, D., Cooper, P. and Day, A (1982). Hysterectomy and psychiatric disorder. I: levels of psychiatric morbidity before and after hysterectomy. *British Journal of Psychiatry*, **140**, 335–42.

Gould, D. (1990). *Nursing Care of Women*. Hemel Hempstead: Prentice Hall.

Greenberg, M. (1983). The meaning of menorrhagia: an investigation into the associations between the complaint of menorrhagia and depression. *Journal of Psychosomatic Research*, **27**, 209–14.

Hart, R. R. (1980). The influence of a taped hypnotic induction treatment procedure on the recovery of surgery patients. *International Journal of Clinical and Experimental Psychology*, **28**, 324–32.

Hathaway, D. (1986). Effects of preoperative instruction on postoperative outcomes: a meta-analysis. *Nursing Research*, **35**, 269–75.

Hufnagel, V. G. (1988). The conspiracy against the uterus. *Journal of Psychosomatic Obstetrics and Gynaecology*, **9**, 51–8.

Hunter, M. (1994). *Counselling in Obstetrics and Gynaecology*. Leicester: British Psychological Society.

Ivins, J. P. and Kent, G. G. (1993). Women's preferences for male or female gynaecologists. *Journal of Reproductive and Infant Psychology*, **11**, 209–14.

Janis, I. L. (1958). *Psychological Stress*. New York: John Wiley and Sons.

Johnston, M. (1980). Anxiety in surgical patients. *Psychological Medicine*, **10**, 145–52.

Johnston, M. (1987). Emotional and cognitive aspects of anxiety in surgical patients. *Communication and Cognition*, **20**, 245–60.

Ludwick-Rosenthal, R. and Neufeld, R. W. J. (1988). Stress management during noxious medical procedures: an evaluative review of outcome studies. *Psychological Bulletin*, **104**, 326–42.

Marteau, T. (1990). Anxieties in women undergoing colposcopy. *British Journal of Obstetrics and Gynaecology*, **97**, 859–61.

Mathews, A. and Ridgeway, V. (1984). Psychological preparation for surgery. In *Health Care and Human Behaviour* (A. Steptoe and A. Mathews, eds). London: Academic Press.

McKie, L. (1993). Women's views of the cervical smear test: implications for nursing practice. *Journal of Advanced Nursing*, **18**, 1228–34.

Melamed, B. G. (1984). Health intervention: collaboration for health and science. In *Psychology and Health*. The Master Lecture Series, vol. 3 (B. L. Hammonds and C. J. Scheirer, eds). Washington DC: American Psychological Association.

Menage, J. (1993). Post-traumatic stress disorder in women who have undergone obstetric and/or gynaecological procedures. A consecutive series of 30 cases of PTSD. *Journal of Reproductive and Infant Psychology*, **11**, 221–8.

Miller, S. M. (1980). When is a little information a dangerous thing? Coping with stressful events by monitoring versus blunting. *Coping and Health*, NATO Conference Series III, vol. 12.

Miller, S. M. (1988). The interacting effects of coping styles and situation variables in gynecologic settings: implications for research and treatment. *Journal of Psychosomatic Obstetrics and Gynaecology*, **9**, 23–34.

Miller, S. M. and Mangan, C. E. (1983). Interacting effects of information and coping style in adaptation to gynaecologic stress: should the doctor tell all? *Journal of Personality and Social Psychology*, **45**, 223–36.

Moore, J. T. and Tolley, D. H. (1976). Depression following hysterectomy. *Psychosomatics*, **17**, 86–9.

Mumford, E., Schlesinger, H. and Glass, G. V. (1982). The effects of psychological intervention for surgery and heart attacks: an analysis of the literature. *American Journal of Public Health*, **72**, 141–51.

Nugent, L. and Tamlyn-Leaman, K. (1992). The colposcopy experience: what do women know? *Journal of Advanced Nursing*, **17**, 514–20.

Oates, M. and Gath, D. (1989). Psychological aspects of gynaecological surgery. *Balliere's Clinical Obstetrics and Gynaecology*, **3**, 729–49.

Patterson, R. M. and Craig, J. B. (1963). Misconceptions concerning the psychological effects of hysterectomy. *American Journal of Obstetrics and Gynaecology*, **85**, 104–11.

Posner, T. and Vesey, M. (1988). *Presentation of Cervical Cancer: The Patients' View*. London: King's Fund.

Quilliam, S. (1989). *Positive Smear*. 2nd edn, London: Charles Letts.

Raphael, M. (1972). The crisis of hysterectomy. *Australia and New Zealand Journal of Psychiatry*, **6**, 106–15.

Reading, A. E. (1982). The effects of psychological preparation on pain and recovery after minor gynaecological surgery: a preliminary report. *Journal of Clinical Psychology*, **38**, 504–12.

Rees, M. (1981). The control of menorrhagia. In *Gynaecology and Nursing Practice* (Shorthouse and Brush, eds). London: Bailliere Tindall.

Richards, D. H. (1973). Depression after hysterectomy. *Lancet*, **ii**, 430–32.

Richards, D. H. (1974). A post-hysterectomy syndrome. *Lancet*, **ii**, 983–5.

Ridgeway, V. and Mathews, A. (1982). Psychological preparation for surgery: a comparison of methods. *British Journal of Clinical Psychology*, **21**, 271–80.

Ryan, M. M., Dennerstein, L. and Pepperell, R. (1989). Psychological aspects of hysterectomy: a prospective study. *British Journal of Psychiatry*, **154**, 516–22.

Scottish Health Statistics (1992). Information and Statistics Division, Common Services Agency for the Scottish Health Service, Edinburgh.

Settlage, D. (1975). Pelvic examinations of women. In Human Needs and Nursing Practice (1982) (J. S. Weinberg, ed.) Philadelphia: W.B. Saunders and Co.

Slade, P., Anderton, K. J. and Faragher, E. B. (1988). Psychological aspects of gynaecological outpatients. Journal of Psychosomatic Obstetrics and Gynaecology, 8, 77–94.

Sloan, D. (1978). The emotional and psychosexual aspects of hysterectomy. Obstetrics and Gynaecology, 131, 598–605.

Spielberger, C. D., Gorsuch, R. L., Lushene, R. E., Vagg, P. R. and Jacobs, G. A. (1983). Manual for the State-Trait Anxiety Inventory (Form Y). Palo Alto, CA: Consulting Psychologists Press Inc.

Steptoe, A. and O'Sullivan, J. (1986). Monitoring and blunting coping styles in women prior to surgery. British Journal of Clinical Psychology, 25, 143–4.

Travis, C. B. (1985). Medical decision making and elective surgery: the case of hysterectomy. Risk Analysis, 5, 241–51.

Wallace, L. M. (1983). Psychological studies of the development and evaluation of preparatory procedures for women undergoing minor gynaecological surgery. University of Birmingham: unpublished PhD thesis.

Wallace, L. M. (1984). Psychological preparation for gynaecological surgery. In Psychology and Gynaecological Problems (A. Broome and L. Wallace, eds). New York: Tavistock.

Wallace, L. M. (1986). Informed consent to elective surgery: the 'therapeutic' value. Social Science and Medicine, 22, 29–33.

Warrington, K. and Gottlieb, L. (1987). Uncertainty and anxiety of hysterectomy during hospitalization. Nursing Papers, 19, 59–73.

Weinman, J. and Johnston, M. (1988). Stressful medical procedures: an analysis of the effects of psychological interventions and of the stressfulness of the procedures. In Topics in Health Psychology (S. Maes, C. D. Spielberger, P. D. Dafares and I. G. Sarason, eds). London: John Wiley and Sons.

Wijma, K. (1984). Psychological functioning after non-cancerous hysterectomy: a review of methods and results. Journal of Psychosomatic Obstetrics and Gynaecology, 3, 133–54.

Wijma, K and Areskog-Wijma, B. (1987). Women's experiences of their genitals as an important aspect of their meetings with gynaecologists. Journal of Psychosomatic Obstetrics and Gynaecology, 6, 133–41.

Wilkinson, C., Jones, J. H. and McBride, J. (1990). Anxiety caused by an abnormal result of cervical smear test: a controlled trial. British Medical Journal, 300, 440.

Williams, S. (1992). Evaluative studies of different forms of communication designed to meet the needs of women with cervical intraepithelial neoplasia. Part 1 Report: knowledge status, anxiety and coping. Greater Glasgow Health Board.

Williams, S. (1994). Information package for women with abnormal cervical smears (letters, leaflets, video and audiotapes). Greater Glasgow Health Board.

Wright, R. C. (1969). Hysterectomy: past present and future. Obstetrics and Gynaecology, 3, 560–63.

# 6

# Andrology: men and reproduction

## Kenneth Gannon

Men are often neglected in discussions of reproduction. Although men are not naturally able to conceive and bear a child, this is not, as this book aims to demonstrate, the beginning and end of human reproduction. Both men and women have reproductive organs and reproductive hormones. Both men and women experience gender, puberty, sexuality, fertility and parenthood. Reproductive potential is a concern for and an influence on men and women. The inclusion of only one chapter in this book explicitly about men and reproduction does not mean that we think that reproduction is less important for men, it simply reflects the dearth of research about men in a culture which labels men as 'productive' while women are 'reproductive'. The research described by Kenneth Gannon in this chapter essentially complements that in Chapter 5. He is concerned with psychosocial aspects of problems and diseases associated with the male reproductive system. A comparison of the two chapters raises some interesting political questions though, such as why are GPs paid to screen women routinely for cervical and breast cancer, but not to screen men for testicular cancer? Why isn't bilateral orchidectomy (removal of the testes) advocated as a prevention for testicular cancer, while ovariectomy is seen as appropriate to prevent ovarian cancer? These questions increase our awareness of the socio-political aspects of human reproduction as well as the psychological aspects, and link us back to the considerations of what male and female mean in Chapter 1.

## Introduction

The male reproductive system consists of:

- left and right testes (the gonads) containing highly coiled tubules within which sperm are produced
- accessory sex glands, including seminal vesicles and the prostate, which produce secretions essential for the normal functioning of the sperm
- external genitalia – the penis and scrotum
- a series of passageways or ducts linking these components.

Andrology is the medical specialization dealing with the morphology and diseases of this highly complex system. This chapter draws together some recent work on the psychosocial aspects of some of these diseases. It does not attempt to provide coverage of the whole range of possible problems. The topics which have been selected for inclusion have been chosen on the basis of three criteria. Firstly, they are problems which affect the capacity to reproduce or the satisfaction derived from sexual activity or both, secondly, they affect substantial numbers of men and, thirdly, a reasonably large body of empirical research was available for review. Four topics met these criteria: cancer of the testis, cancer of the prostate, benign prostatic hypertrophy and sexual dysfunction. Male infertility, although it met the above criteria, has not been included as it will be dealt with in a separate volume.

While the specialism of gynaecology has seen a growing awareness of the importance of considering the role of psychosocial factors in understanding phenomena and conditions as diverse as chronic pelvic pain, the menstrual cycle, gynaecological cancer, contraception and hysterectomy, very little has been written about the psychosocial aspects of andrological conditions and disorders. This is clear from the relatively small number of research papers published in the area. For example, a search of the psychological literature for the period 1987–1993 identified 24 papers which made reference to the psychological aspects of testicular cancer and 13 dealing with psychological aspects of cancer of the prostate. A search covering the same period for psychological aspects of breast cancer identified 326 papers. (A similar search of the biomedical literature published during the same period yielded 35 and 33 papers dealing with testicular and prostatic cancer respectively compared to 478 papers relating to breast cancer.) Such an imbalance suggests both that the study of psychosocial aspects of disorders of the male reproductive system is in its infancy and that many issues are likely to be unresolved, if indeed they have even been addressed. That this is indeed the case will become clear in the following reviews.

## Cancer of the testis

Testicular cancer accounts for 1 per cent of all male malignancies. Although relatively rare it is the most common type of cancer in men aged 15 to 35 (Vogt and McHale, 1992). The incidence of testicular tumours has been rising for the last forty years in the West, current incidence figures are 3.8 per 100 000 in England and Wales (Williams, 1990) and 2.1 per 100 000 in the US (Moynihan, 1991). This type of cancer is more common in men of higher socio-economic groups (Williams, 1990).

The majority of patients present with a testicular swelling which is usually painless. Other symptoms include a heavy sensation in the scrotum, breast enlargement and tenderness and back pain (Vogt and McHale, 1992).

The initial treatment is generally surgical removal of the affected testicle, a procedure known as radical orchidectomy. Subsequent treatment is determined by histologic results and the stage of the disease and may involve radiotherapy, chemotherapy or, in certain instances, removal of enlarged lymph glands in the abdomen. This latter procedure is known as retroperitoneal lymph node dissection (RPLND). This may involve sacrifice of the sympathetic nerve plexus which can jeopardize normal sexual function and lead to impotence or retrograde ejaculation (Vogt and McHale, 1992).

Despite the increasing incidence of this type of cancer mortality rates are improving because of successful treatment. While in the 1950s half the men in whom testicular cancer had spread to other sites in the body died within three years of diagnosis, recent reports indicate cure rates of between 70 per cent and 90 per cent, depending on the type of tumour and the degree of progression of the disease (Williams, 1990; Moynihan, 1991). A consequence of this is that many young men are surviving and having to come to terms with a range of psychosocial issues relating to the nature of the disease itself and the consequences of the treatment employed. These issues will be described and discussed under a number of headings.

## Sexual functioning

The effects of treatment on sexual functioning are complex and are to some extent treatment specific. They also vary depending on the parameters of sexual function which are measured. Treatments such as RPLND which interfere with autonomic inervation generally seem to result in higher rates of sexual dysfunction. Combining RPLND with additional treatments such as radiotherapy and chemotherapy may lead to higher rates of specific problems, such as a reduction in orgasmic intensity (Tross, 1989).

Many men report reduced levels of sexual activity following treatment. Schover and von Eschenbach (1985) compared a group of young men who had undergone RPLND with a similar group of healthy men. The treatment group reported lower levels of sexual activity; 11 per cent of this group compared with 0 per cent in the comparison group reported no current sexual activity.

Treated men who remain sexually active report reductions in measures of sexual performance and pleasure. Common problems are erectile dysfunction, difficulty in achieving orgasm, reduced intensity of orgasm, dry ejaculations, reduced semen volume and generally reduced satisfaction with sex. Overall rates of sexual dysfunction are in the range 10–50 per cent (Tross, 1989; Moynihan, 1991). Such problems are more common in groups treated for testicular cancer than in healthy men. Sexual problems are often highly interrelated. For example, Schover, Gonzales and von Eschenbach (1986) found highly significant relationships between erectile dysfunction and difficulty reaching orgasm and between reduced semen volume and reduced orgasmic pleasure. Sexual dysfunction and anxiety about fertility are also related, Rieker, Edbril and Garnick (1985) found a highly significant association between ejaculatory dysfunction and infertility distress. The severity of these various dysfunctions is related both to the nature and the extent of treatment (Schover and von Eschenbach, 1985).

There is some evidence of a relationship between the degree of sexual dysfunction and psychological factors, although the direction of the relationship has yet to be established. Rieker, Edbril and Garnick (1985) reported that men who tended to conceal their emotions had higher sexual impairment scores than those who expressed them. In a subsequent study Rieker, Fitzgerald, Kalish et al., (1989) reported that scores for negative mental outlook (reflecting negative attitudes to the future) were higher among men with sexual dysfunction than among those without (26 per cent versus 13 per cent).

## Relationships and self-image

There is no evidence to suggest that marital relationships are more likely to fail following diagnosis and treatment of testicular cancer. Several studies (e.g. Schover and von Eschenbach, 1985; Rieker, Edbril and Garnick, 1985) have reported divorce rates no different from those of a similar group of healthy men. There is some evidence that lover relationships are more vulnerable to strain (Rieker, Edbril and Garnick, 1985) as are those which were unhappy prior to the diagnosis of cancer (Schover, Gonzales and von Eschenbach, 1986). There may, in fact, be a positive effect on relationships. Rieker, Edbril and Garnick (1985) found that 68 per cent of married men reported that their relationship with their spouse was strengthened, while Hannah, Gritz, Wellisch et al., (1992), in a comparison of long-term survivors of testicular cancer and Hodgkin's Disease, found that similar proportions of both groups (83.3 per cent) reported that the illness had drawn them closer together. Although many men report a decline in sexual satisfaction, their spouses may be more happy than before; Gritz, Wellisch, Wang et al., (1989) found that 47.1 per cent of the spouses reported increased sexual satisfaction. They speculated that this 'silver lining effect' may have been a product of an increased intimacy resulting from deepened bonds due to shared adversity.

Many studies have found enhanced life satisfaction following treatment. Rieker, Edbril and Garnick (1985), for example, reported that the majority of men felt that the cancer experience had improved their lives, particularly in terms of outlook on life and relationship with children, although some areas, notably satisfaction with sex and ability to be active, had become worse.

Cassileth and Steinfeld (1987) found no differences between a patient and a control group in terms of perceptions of their own masculinity following treatment. Gritz, Wellisch, Wang et al., (1989) reported that the majority of patients (64.7 per cent) and spouses (88.2 per cent) did not perceive a decrease in overall attractiveness as a result of treatment.

### Fertility issues

Prior to excision of the affected testicle approximately 50 per cent of men with testicular cancer will have below average sperm counts. Following unilateral orchidectomy but before radiotherapy 50–79 per cent of men will have abnormally low sperm counts. Immediately following radiotherapy most men will not be producing sperm (azoospermic) although spermatogenesis often recovers within 1–5 years. Several studies have found that the majority of men who wanted to father a child following treatment were able to do so. No excess of birth defects has been reported in the resulting children (Tross, 1989; Moynihan, 1991).

Despite these encouraging findings there is evidence that anxiety regarding fertility status is an issue for men following treatment. Rieker, Fitzgerald, Kalish et al., (1989) reported that 22 per cent of men in their study reported high distress about possible loss of fertility. Higher rates of distress were seen among younger, childless, less educated men of lower income and lower occupational status. Such anxiety is likely to be exacerbated by some of the consequences of treatment. Schover and von Eschenbach (1985) reported that in a group of 121 men 56.9 per cent experienced 'dry' orgasm and that overall the volume of semen was greatly reduced in 82.1 per cent of men. Many men bank sperm prior to treatment but there is no evidence that those who do so experience lower levels of anxiety regarding infertility (Rieker, Edbril and Garnick, 1985).

### Early detection of testicular cancer

The prognosis for testicular cancer is good particularly if detected early, yet many men delay before seeking medical advice following the appearance of symptoms. The mean delay is in the range fourteen (Jones and Appleyard, 1989) to twenty-one weeks (Moul, Paulson, Dodge et al., 1990). Studies have reported an association between consultation delay, increased stage of disease and lowered probability of survival in several types of testicular tumour (Moul, Paulson, Dodge et al., 1990). Principal causes of delay appear to be ignorance, embarrassment, fear of cancer and fear of emasculation (Post and Belis, 1980; Jones and Appleyard, 1989). Many efforts to reduce the delay to consultation have focused on health education. Surveys have found low levels of knowledge both about the nature, risks and presentation of testicular cancer and low rates of carrying out testicular self-examination (TSE) which is necessary for the detection of symptoms. Sheley, Kinchen and Morgan et al., (1991) surveyed 415 men in New Orleans and Rochester, New York. Only 2 per cent of respondents reported carrying out monthly TSE at the correct time and with the proper method. Klein, Berry and Felice (1990) surveyed a group of sixty-six 15–20 year olds. Fifteen per cent were aware of the risks of testicular cancer. No one was able to describe the symptoms of testicular cancer and only 1.5 per cent reported regularly carrying out TSE. Docks, Garb, White et al., (1989) found that of 633 students in three New England colleges 4.7 per cent performed monthly TSE.

Intervention strategies have been designed to increase rates of TSE. Klein, Berry and Felice (1990) gave a programmed, self-instruction booklet on TSE to their study group of adolescents. At a two-year follow-up 67 per cent reported performing regular TSE and 95 per cent knew that a small lump was the most common symptom of testicular cancer. Murphy and Brubaker (1990) reported that a group who had received information about testicular cancer and TSE, and a message challenging negative beliefs about TSE were more likely to perform TSE subsequently than a control group.

## Issues and future directions

As the incidence and survival rates of testicular cancer continue to increase, the need to take account of the psychosocial aspects of the disease becomes more pressing. The present review indicates some approaches which may be helpful.

To date most of the cohorts of survivors studied have been heterogeneous with respect to the length of time since treatment was completed, with periods ranging from one year to twenty years. There is a need to evaluate more homogeneous groups and identify more clearly those factors indicative of a poor prognosis and those associated with effective coping. The fact that most sufferers tend to be from the higher social classes and to be better educated than is the case in other cancers means that there is a degree of confounding between these variables and coping and adjustment; this needs to be clarified. The same applies to a confound between anxiety levels and their possible relation to the duration, extent or type of treatment and measures of sexual satisfaction and performance.

Early detection is clearly a crucial factor in successful treatment and while interventions to increase the rates of TSE have produced promising results there remain a number of unresolved issues. The dependent measure in most studies is self-reported rates of compliance. The accuracy of self-report is open to doubt (e.g. Ley, 1988) and therefore reported increases in compliance must, at this stage, be regarded with caution. Furthermore, there is no evidence as yet on whether these interventions have had an impact on delay to consultation in cases where a suspicious lump was detected. As the intention of such programmes is to detect cancers at a sufficiently early stage to prevent their spread to other sites in the body it is clearly important to demonstrate that not only do participants carry out TSE but that they act on any suspicious findings. It may be that, in order to lead to such outcomes, programmes designed to increase rates of TSE need to be combined with others designed to deal with the causes of delay out-lined above, such as embarrassment and fear. No such combined programmes appear to have been evaluated as yet.

The relatively high levels of sexually-related problems and anxiety in this group suggest the need for ready availability of support and counselling services, both for individuals and for couples. A particular problem, recognized by those working with sufferers from testicular cancer, is that men in the greatest need may not seek psychological support and, as noted above, there is a tendency for such men to conceal their emotions. As yet no systematic evaluation of psycho-logical therapy with this group has been published but psychological therapies have shown promise with other groups of cancer sufferers and may well have an important role to play in this area also. An example is Adjuvant Psychological Therapy (APT), a brief, problem-focused therapy which is based on Beck's cognitive approach to therapy. It is designed to encourage the expression of feelings, promote a sense of control, help clients to develop coping strategies and improve communication between the patient and their partner (Moorey and Greer, 1989; Moorey, 1991). APT has been reported to reduce anxiety and depression, increase fighting spirit and reduce helplessness in individuals suffering from a variety of cancers (Moorey, 1991).

# Cancer of the prostate

In England and Wales prostatic cancer is the third most frequent cause of deaths due to malignancies, while in men it is second only to lung cancer (Williams, 1990). In the US it is the most common malignancy affecting men and is third, behind lung and colon cancer, as a cause of male cancer deaths (Kemp, 1992). It is uncommon before 50 years of age but its incidence increases extremely rapidly thereafter (Williams, 1990). The most frequent early presenting symptom is difficulty with passing urine. Advanced presentation includes bladder obstruction with urine retention, urethral obstruction, renal failure and weight loss and anorexia (Williams, 1990; Kemp, 1992). The treatments employed are surgical removal of the prostate (radical prostatectomy), radiotherapy and hormonal therapy, which may include orchidectomy in advanced cases to prevent stimulation of tumour growth by testosterone. Each of these treatments has side effects associated with it (Williams, 1990).

## Screening

As is the case with other types of malignancy the prognosis in cases of prostate cancer is markedly improved if treatment is initiated before local or distant spread (Kemp, 1992). A particular problem is that symptoms develop late; autopsy studies have demonstrated unsuspected disease in 5–10 per cent of men at age 50 (Kemp, 1992). There is some debate as to whether the currently avail-able screening methods meet the criteria for effective screening (Kemp, 1992). Notwithstanding these problems efforts are being made to screen for carcinoma of the prostate in at-risk populations. The most commonly employed form of initial screening is digital rectal examination, although transrectal ultrasound (TRUS) examination is becoming more widely employed. In cases of suspected malignancy a fine needle aspiration biopsy is performed (Kemp, 1992).

Chadwick, Kemple, Astley et al., (1991) carried out a study of screening in general practice, the main aim being to assess the patient acceptability of such a procedure. All men on the practice list aged between 55 and 70 were contacted. Screening consisted of measurement of serum prostate specific antigen (PSA) and digital rectal examination. Patients who met specified criteria were referred for transrectal ultrasonography. The overall recruitment was 58 per cent (472 from a population of 814) and no patient who attended refused PSA measurement. A few refused digital rectal examination and of seventy-five men referred for transrectal ultrasonography six declined. The authors concluded that these low rejection rates indicated that the process was acceptable to the patients.

Pederson, Carlsson, Varenhorst et al., (1990) carried out a similar study in Sweden. They randomly selected 1494 from a population of 9026 men aged between 50 and 69 years, of whom 1163 (78 per cent) attended. The highest acceptance rate was among men aged 60–64. Of the 331 who declined to attend 142 were anxious or sceptical about the programme and 189 gave other reasons, such as being under medical care already. Data were gathered on the distress experienced by the patients. Immediately after digital rectal examination patients were asked about discomfort during the exam and patients referred for biopsy completed questionnaires immediately following the procedure about mental stress during the preceding week and physical discomfort during the procedure. They completed another stress questionnaire after they received the results of the biopsy. Most men experienced no distress during the first examination, although there was a slight tendency for younger men to report more distress than older ones. Of the forty-four men who were recalled on suspicion of malignancy twenty-five were anxious during the week of waiting and eighteen were more nervous than usual. Thirty one felt anxious while awaiting the report and most were unusually nervous. These authors also concluded that the screening method is acceptable to the patients and is not unduly uncomfortable.

Collins, Lloyd, Hehir et al., (1993) carried out a study focusing specifically on patient acceptance of prostatic biopsies carried out via the rectum and guided by means of ultrasound. Following the procedure and before discharge from the clinic all eighty-nine patients received a questionnaire about the procedure which they were requested to return within one week. The vast majority of patients reported satisfaction with the explanation provided, 22 per cent found the procedure painful, 68 per cent experienced mild discomfort and 10 per cent experienced no discomfort. Forty per cent felt embarrassed during the procedure, 3 per cent extremely so.

Although there appears to be a consensus that current screening procedures are acceptable to the target population no studies have been conducted of men's knowledge of symptoms of prostatic carcinoma or of the incidence and course of the condition. It is not clear, therefore, whether men are likely to seek consultation on their own initiative or whether the onus must be on physicians to screen at-risk populations.

## Effects of treatment

The treatment of choice for prostatic cancer depends on its stage. Many clinicians regard orchidectomy as the initial treatment of choice for advanced prostatic cancer while radical prostatectomy may be selected for a localized tumour (Williams, 1990; Kemp, 1992). All forms of treatment of prostatic cancer have been reported to cause sexual dysfunction, although the frequency of dysfunction varies with the method of treatment and the particular study. The effects of diagnostic and treatment procedures on sexual function have been studied since the late 1950s, although it is only relatively recently that researchers have attempted to address the psychological effects. These recent studies have tended to focus on the patient acceptability of particular procedures and on their psychological impact.

Parmar, Phillips, Lightman et al., (1985) addressed the issue of impact by randomly allocating patients with advanced prostatic carcinoma either to an orchidectomy (thirty-eight patients) or a drug treatment group (forty-one patients). The drug employed acted to reduce hormone levels and thus had an effect similar to orchidectomy. For this reason such treatment is sometimes referred to as 'medical orchidectomy' or 'medical castration'. Patients completed questionnaires relating to pain and mood states both before treatment and at follow-up in outpatients. Before treatment there were no differences between the groups on mood score. However, at six-month follow-up patients in the drug group tended to have less fatigue, anger, depression and anxiety and to be more cheerful and energetic than the orchidectomy patients, although these differences did not achieve statistical significance. Both groups were equal on pain scores before treatment and similar numbers in each showed a reduction in pain score following treatment. These results were replicated in a subsequent study (Parmar, Edwards, Phillips et al., 1987).

Parmar, Phillips, Edwards et al., (1988) reported that they subsequently informed the patients who participated in their earlier studies about the clinical results of surgical and medical orchidectomy. About 70 per cent of those from the surgical group said that they would select medical orchidectomy given the choice while all of the patients receiving the drug preferred to continue to receive it as long as they were in remission. This finding suggests that while no studies have reported significant levels of distress due to orchidectomy, patients may come to regret an irreversible surgical procedure.

In a study of patient choice Chadwick, Kemple and Astley et al., (1991) informed patients that they had cancer of the prostate and gave them details of both of the treatment options available (orchidectomy and drug treatment) and the associated side effects. Of the fifty patients interviewed twenty-three chose to undergo orchidectomy and twenty-seven to receive the drug. The reasons given for choosing the drug included avoidance both of the operation itself and of possible delays in surgery due to waiting lists. Reasons given for choosing orchidectomy included avoidance of continued regular hospital visits and the consequent disruption of daily life. The two groups did not differ in age or disease stage although more inpatients chose the surgical option.

Moore, O'Sullivan and Tannock (1988) asked physicians what treatment they would choose for themselves if they had localized prostate cancer. Of those sampled, 39 per cent opted for radiotherapy and 40 per cent for radical prostatectomy. When offered the hypothetical opportunity to participate in a randomized trial comparing these two therapies, 71 per cent of urologists rejected the trial because they felt that surgery was superior, while none rejected the trial because they felt that radiotherapy was superior.

In the case of localized tumours the different treatment options may have different associated costs, in terms of the risk of impotence, and benefits, in terms of probability of survival. This raises the issue of whether men may be prepared to make a trade-off between quality and quantity of life. Singer, Tasch, Stocking et al., (1991) addressed this by interviewing fifty men aged between 45 and 70 years without known prostatic cancer and asking them to choose between a series of combinations of chance of surviving for five years and probability of potency. They found that, within limits, men may be willing (in a hypothetical situation at least) to trade off survival in order to increase their chances of remaining sexually potent.

### Issues and future directions

There is a clear need for greater research emphasis on the psychosocial and psychosexual consequences of cancer of the prostate taking into account age-related factors and pre-morbidity levels of sexual activity. The effects of treatments, including the issue of patient choice, also require further study. Such studies as have been carried out have been marred by a failure to employ a consistent set of standardized psychological assessments and a failure to provide comparison or control groups. There is also a need for a study to evaluate the efficacy of psychologically-based interventions with this group.

## Benign prostatic hypertrophy (BPH)

Benign enlargement (hypertrophy) of the prostate occurs to some extent in all men after middle age. It becomes a cause for concern only when the enlargement obstructs the flow of urine leading to difficulties in urination and, in severe cases, to acute urine retention. This obstruction occurs because the urethra passes through the centre of the prostate after leaving the bladder and as the prostate enlarges it squeezes the urethra, making urination difficult or even impossible. Symptoms of obstruction include the need to urinate frequently, often accompanied by a feeling of urgency, frequent waking in order to urinate (nocturia), poor flow of urine and difficulty in initiating urination. In such cases surgical removal of part or all of the gland to relieve the obstruction (prostatectomy) may be required. This form of treatment is required in approximately 10 per cent of cases (Blandy, 1989). Several surgical options are available, but nowadays in all but cases of men with very large prostates the standard procedure is transurethral resection of the prostate (TURP). This involves the insertion of an instrument called a resectoscope via the penis. The obstructing prostatic tissue is then cut away by a heated wire loop contained in the resectoscope. Approximately 31 000 such procedures are conducted annually in England (Lynch, Waymont, Beacock et al., 1991).

### Effects of TURP on health and well-being

There are a number of possible side effects associated with prostatectomy. These can be divided into two broad classes, effects on continence and effects on sexual function.

Urinary incontinence is a rare but extremely distressing complication of prostatectomy. It is estimated to occur in two out of every 1000 cases treated by means of TURP in the United States (Kaufman, 1986).

Prostatectomy can influence sexual function in a variety of ways, through its effects on potency and ejaculatory function. Unlike radical prostatectomy which, prior to the development of procedures which avoided damage to the nerves involved in sexual functioning, frequently resulted in impotence, resection of the prostate rarely has a severe impact in this respect. Nevertheless, problems can occur and attempts have been made to reduce them. Zohar, Meiraz, Maoz et al., (1976) interviewed fifteen patients prior to prostatectomy and again six months postoperatively. Seven of these patients were given an explanation of the operation prior to surgery. This covered details of the procedure and reassurances that preoperative sexual capacity would be maintained despite the dry orgasm. Of the seven who received the explanation none reported impotence six months post-operatively while of the eight who did not receive it five became impotent and two complained of disturbances in sexual function.

The neck of the bladder is removed by prostatectomy, so the bladder is no longer shut off from the prostatic cavity during ejaculation and semen can pass back into the bladder. Some degree of this so-called retrograde (dry) ejaculation occurs commonly both after open prostatectomy and TURP and may be a source of considerable anxiety to some men. The rates of this disturbance vary from study to study. Hargreave and Stephenson (1977) reported that 54 per cent of patients had total retrograde ejaculation following TURP, while Newman, Reiss and Northup (1982) reported a rate of 30 per cent. Retrograde ejaculation means that normal fertilization is impossible and may thus be a cause of anxiety in men who wish to father a child. Additionally, anxiety over the nature of the orgasm itself may be a source of distress. The study of Zohar, Meiraz, Maoz et al., (1976) demonstrates the importance of good communication in this respect.

The pre- and post-operative symptomatology and health status of a large cohort of men (398) undergoing TURP has been extensively studied by Doll and her colleagues (Doll, Black, McPherson et al., 1992, Doll, Black, Flood et al., 1993a and b). The most common symptoms experienced by these men before surgery were poor stream, dribbling, frequency and nocturia (85–95 per cent). These symptoms were reported to affect sexual activity (31 per cent of the respondents), social activities (29 per cent) and holidays (29 per cent). After surgery, 60–78 per cent of patients reported improvements in prostate-related symptoms or health problems (Doll, Black, Flood et al., 1993a and b). Nevertheless, 38 per cent reported urinary incontinence for at least two weeks postoperatively and, at three months 20 per cent were still incontinent. At the three-month stage 44 per cent of the patients reported either incontinence or urinary tract infection, although this had dropped to 12 per cent at one year (Doll, Black, McPherson et al., 1992). However, only 6 per cent of the men reported an improvement in their sex lives, with 25 per cent reporting a deterioration (Doll, Black, McPherson et al., 1992). The pre- and post-operative prevalences of impotence were similar. Men who were impotent before the operation were more likely to be impotent one year afterwards than those who were not

The majority of men who undergo prostatectomy, particularly TURP, appear to be satisfied with the outcome of the procedure and to be in good health. Nevertheless, a substantial minority report a deterioration in sexual function and it seems important to determine whether this may be predicted pre-operatively and whether it can be avoided or remedied in any way. Similarly, while the health impact of the procedure seems generally positive some men report symptoms which adversely affect their quality of life. Again, such men need to be identified and offered help. The reproductive implications of the procedure for younger men also require further study.

## Male sexual dysfunction

The identification of male sexual dysfunction is related to the understanding of normal function. Kaplan (1974, 1977) identified three categories of disorder related to the stages of sexual arousal. The first stage, sexual desire, includes hypoactive and hyperactive desire disorders. The second phase, sexual excitement, includes erectile disorders (impotence) and the third phase, orgasm, includes premature and retarded ejaculation. It is usual to draw a further distinction between primary (present since puberty) and secondary (following a period of normal functioning) disorders in addition to considering whether the disorder is pervasive or situational. Most authors favour a multifactorial model of causation, emphasizing the interaction of psychological, physiological, environmental and relationship factors (e.g. Masters and Johnson, 1970; Kaplan, 1974). A range of specific factors should also be considered. These include ignorance about sexual function (Bancroft, 1989), negative or overly moralistic attitudes (Masters and Johnson, 1970), anxiety about sexual performance (Bancroft, 1989), spectatoring (tendency to observe oneself during sexual activity; Masters and Johnson, 1970), and a range of physical problems such as diabetes, neurological damage, drug use and ageing. Approaches to therapy are described in Masters and Johnson, (1970); Kaplan, (1974); de Silva, (1987) and Bancroft (1989), among others. Commonly employed treatments include couples therapy, desensitization, hormonal treatments, surgically implanted mechanical prostheses designed to produce an erection and psychotherapy. The selection of a particular intervention depends largely on the nature of the disorder.

Erectile dysfunction (ED) has been a particular focus of interest from both theoretical and clinical perspectives and for this reason has been selected for discussion in this chapter. Erectile dysfunction has been identified as a common problem both in surveys of the general population and in studies conducted in medical settings, such as general practice (Slag, Morley, Elson et al., 1983; Spector and Boyle, 1986). Men suffering from ED produce smaller erections and show a longer latency to achieve erections than comparison groups (Kockott, Feil, Ferstl et al., 1980; Heiman and Rowland, 1983; Beck and Barlow, 1986). Erectile dysfunction was thought to be due largely to psychogenic factors, such as performance anxiety and spectatoring, but in recent research greater recognition is being given to the role of organic factors, such as side effects of medication and neurological problems (Slag, Morley, Elson et al., 1983; Melman, Tiefer and Pederson, 1988; Speckens, Hengeveld, Lycklama a Nijeholt et al., 1993). Attempts are usually made to identify the principal aetiological factor early in assessment. This is done in order to guide the selection both of further tests and of the most appropriate therapy.

One of the most widely used diagnostic techniques has been nocturnal penile tumescence monitoring (NPT). The rationale underlying this procedure is that if spontaneous erections occur during sleep then it is unlikely that an organic problem is present. However, a number of authors have begun to question its reliability (e.g. Meisler and Carey, 1990) and because of this and also because the equipment necessary to perform this assessment is not always routinely available, attempts have been made to utilize standardized psychometric instruments to discriminate organic from psychogenic ED. Beutler, Karacan, Anch et al., (1975) utilized the Minnesota Multiphasic Personality Inventory

(MMPI) to distinguish between the two, but subsequent studies have failed to replicate their success (e.g. Levenson, Olkin, Herzoff et al., 1986). Other authors have focused on evaluation of sexual functioning as a possible discriminator. Derogatis, Meyer and Dupkin (1976) employed the Derogatis Sexual Functioning Inventory and reported a correct classification rate of 89 per cent. Once again, however, later studies failed to replicate these findings (e.g. Segraves, Schoenberg, Zairns et al., 1981). Rather better results have been obtained employing questionnaires which examine the sexual symptomatology of ED. Kockott, Feil, Ferstl et al., (1980) distinguished men with psychogenic ED from men with organic ED on the basis of six out of eighty questions on sexual history and Segraves, Segraves and Schoenberg (1987) concluded that the presence of adequate early morning erections, masturbatory erections and non-coital erections discriminated between those with organic and those with psychogenic ED. More recently Speckens, Hengeveld, Lycklama a Nijeholt et al., (1993) demonstrated that responses on the Leiden Impotence Questionnaire enabled correct classification of cases as either psychogenic or organic in 62 per cent and 86 per cent of cases respectively. In many ways the distinction between organic and psychogenic factors is probably artificial, with both contributing in differing proportions in individual cases.

Other studies have focused on the psychological consequences and correlates of sexual dysfunction, primarily ED. A series of investigations have demonstrated that the emotional response of men with a sexual dysfunction to sexual situations is generally characterized by anxiety (e.g. Kockott, Feil, Ferstl et al., 1980; Heiman and Rowland, 1983; Beck and Barlow, 1986). Rowland and Heiman (1991) reported that men suffering from ED showed significantly higher scores on measures of anxiety and depression than did members of a control group. Nevertheless, some studies (e.g. Beck and Barlow, 1986) have suggested that anxiety may not be a contributory factor to sexual dysfunction in all cases. It has been suggested that excessive self-monitoring of genital response at the expense of stimuli from the partner or from fantasy is a contributing factor to psychogenic sexual dysfunction (e.g. Beck, Barlow and Sakheim, 1983; Sakheim, Barlow, Beck et al., 1984). Rowland and Heiman (1991) have reported on a study in which changes in genital arousal (measured by means of a strain gauge) and self-reported arousal (measured by means of visual analogue scales) to erotic stimulation were measured in a group of sexually dysfunctional men before and after a course of sex therapy and compared with those of a control group. Each group was studied under two sets of conditions; one in which the instructions elicited performance demand (focus on the need to satisfy the partner), and one in which they elicited sensate focus (attention on physical sensations). The control group showed enhanced genital response under performance demand conditions while the dysfunctional subjects showed inhibited genital responses. This finding supports the traditional view of anxiety hindering the performance of sexually dysfunctional men. In addition, however, Rowland and Heiman reported a discrepancy between measures of dysfunctional men's self-reported and genital measures of arousal. Self-reported arousal was higher under performance demand conditions than under sensate focus while genital response was slightly lower. The authors speculated that this pattern was indicative of the cognitive distortion which results from excessive self-monitoring and an over-responsiveness to genital cues in situations which involve performance demands. This study also provided evidence for the efficacy of sex therapy in that sexually dysfunctional men showed a greater erectile response to erotic stimulation following sex therapy.

Two points of particular note emerge from this discussion. First, the evidence for the efficacy of sex therapy in treating sexual dysfunction is ambiguous. Although Rowland and Heiman (1991) found some evidence of improved responsiveness in a laboratory test post therapy, the authors themselves acknowledged that this may not necessarily reflect functioning with a sexual partner. Some reports have suggested that coital success may spontaneously improve without intervention (Killman, Milan, Bowland et al., 1987). There is a clear need for further research in this area. Second, the constituent elements of the sexual response are clearly complex and imperfectly correlated, as evidenced by the disjunction of self-reported and erectile responses in Rowland and Heiman's (1991) study. This finding suggests that the nature of the sexual response may differ in functional and dysfunctional men. This indicates a need both to clarify these differences and the factors underlying them and to delineate the stimuli affecting sexual responsivity in dysfunctional men.

## General conclusions

Reviewers frequently conclude their task with a call for more research. While in many cases this may appear overcautious or noncommittal in the present case it can be made with a considerable degree of justification. As noted at the beginning of the chapter, there is a very small body of research on normal functioning for either sex and a still smaller literature on the psychosocial aspects of 'men's problems' compared to that on 'women's problems'. One can only speculate on possible reasons for this state of affairs and consideration of possible explanations, such as male unwillingness to confront the emotional aspects of these disorders, would require chapters in their own right. It is, however, possible to be more specific about some of the issues which could be addressed in future research.

Within the traditional science paradigm, there is a need for more standardized measures to be employed across diagnostic categories in order to identify common patterns of reactions. Within diagnostic categories there is a need to identify more homogeneous groups of individuals and to carry out longitudinal, prospective studies of these in order to identify changes in concerns, issues and coping strategies over time.

From a psychosocial perspective, it is clear that although many men and their partners cope well with the difficulties which may arise, others do not. It is important to be able to identify those potentially at risk for negative reactions in order to provide appropriate counselling and support services. Linked to this is the need to evaluate the efficacy of psychological therapies in helping individuals to cope with disorders such as cancer of the prostate. Once again, it would be important to be able to identify those particularly at risk and, crucially, to develop methods of involving them in such programmes.

Overall, there is no information on cultural or ethnic variations in reactions to or methods of coping with these disorders. Coupled with this is a heterosexist bias in the research. Both of these omissions should be rectified in future research.

# Applications

**1. Involve the partner**
Most men cope much better than might be expected with traumatic events such as the loss of a testicle. Support from a partner or spouse is an important factor in this, so steps should be taken to involve them from an early stage in assessment and treatment.

**2. Give information**
Zohar, Meiraz, Maoz et al., (1976) have demonstrated improved outcomes for patients given complete information about each stage of assessment and treatment. This suggests that men and their partners should be told as much as possible about the procedures and possible side effects they will experience.

**3. Improve access to psychological help**
The success of psychological therapies with other forms of cancer suggests that sufferers from andrological cancers and prostate problems would benefit from access to them. Even following successful medical/surgical treatment many men continue to experience psychosocial and health-related problems which may benefit from professional help. Access to such help should continue to be available after medical treatment is completed.

## Further reading

Pryor, J. P. and Lipschulz, L. J. (eds) (1987). *Andrology*. London: Butterworth.
Taguchi, Y. (1988). *Private Parts: A Health Book for Men*. London: Macdonald.
Tanagho, E. A., Lue, T. F. and McClure, R. D. (1988). *Contemporary Management of Impotence and Infertility*. Baltimore: Williams and Wilkins.
Watson, M. (ed.) (1991). *Cancer Patient Care: Psychosocial Treatment Methods*. Leicester: The British Psychological Society.

## References

Bancroft, J. (1989). *Human Sexuality and Its Problems*. 2nd edn, Edinburgh: Churchill Livingstone.
Beck, J. G. and Barlow, D. H. (1986). Effects of anxiety and attentional focus on sexual responding – 1: physiological patterns and erectile dysfunction. *Behavior Research and Therapy*, **24**, 9–17.
Beck, J. G., Barlow, D. H. and Sakheim, D. K. (1983). The effects of attentional focus and partner arousal on sexual responding in functional and dysfunctional men. *Behavior Research and Therapy*, **21**, 1–8.

Beutler, L. E., Karacan, I., Anch, A. M. et al. (1975). MMPI and MIT discriminators of biogenic and psychogenic impotence. *Journal of Consulting and Clinical Psychology*, **43**, 899–903.

Blandy, J. (1989). Prostatic enlargement. *The Practitioner*, **28**, 512–17.

Cassileth, B. R. and Steinfeld, A. D. (1987). Psychological preparation of the patient and family. *Cancer*, **60**, 547–52.

Chadwick, D. J., Kemple, T., Astley, J. P. et al. (1991). Pilot study of screening for prostate cancer in general practice. *Lancet*, **338**, 613–16.

Collins, G. N., Lloyd, S. N., Hehir, M. et al. (1993). Multiple transrectal ultrasound-guided biopsies – true morbidity and patient acceptance. *British Journal of Urology*, **71**, 460–63.

Derogatis, L. R., Meyer, J. K. and Dupkin, C. N. (1976). Discrimination of organic versus psychogenic impotence with the DSFI. *Journal of Sex and Marital Therapy*, **2**, 229–40.

deSilva, P. (1987). Sexual dysfunction: treatment. In *A Handbook of Clinical Adult Psychology* (S. J. E. Lindsay and G. E. Powell, eds) pp. 197–212. Aldershot: Gower.

Docks, R. J., Garb, J. L., White, C. et al. (1989). Male college students compliance with testicular self-examination. *Journal of Adolescent Health Care*, **10**, 295–9.

Doll, H. A., Black, N. A., McPherson, K. et al. (1992). Mortality, morbidity and complications following transurethral resection of the prostate for benign prostatic hypertrophy. *Journal of Urology*, **147**, 1566–73.

Doll, H. A., Black, N. A., Flood, A. B. et al. (1993a). Patient-perceived health status before and up to 12 months after transurethral resection of the prostate for benign prostatic hypertrophy. *British Journal of Urology*, **71**, 297–305.

Doll, H. A., Black, N. A., Flood, A. B. et al. (1993b). Criterion validation of the Nottingham Health Profile: patient views of surgery for benign prostatic hypertrophy. *Social Science and Medicine*, **37**, 115–22.

Gritz, E. R., Wellisch, D. K., Wang, H.-J. et al. (1989). Long-term effects of testicular cancer on sexual functioning in married couples. *Cancer*, **64**, 1560–67.

Hannah, M. T., Gritz, E. R., Wellisch, D. K. et al. (1992). Changes in marital and sexual functioning in long-term survivors and their spouses: Testicular cancer versus Hodgkin's Disease. *Psycho-Oncology*, **1**, 89–103.

Hargreave, T. B. and Stephenson, T. P. (1977). Potency and prostatectomy. *British Journal of Urology*, **49**, 683–8.

Heiman, J. R. and Rowland, D. L. (1983). Affective and physiological response patterns: the effects of instructions on sexually functional and dysfunctional men. *Journal of Psychosomatic Research*, **27**, 105–16.

Jones, W. and Appleyard, I. (1989). Early diagnosis of testicular cancer. *The Practitioner*, **233**, 509–11.

Kaplan, H. S. (1974). *The New Sex Therapy: Brief Treatment of Sexual Dysfunction*. New York: Brunner/Mazel.

Kaplan, H. S. (1977). Hypoactive sexual desire. *Journal of Sex and Marital Therapy*, **3**, 3–9.

Kaufman, J. J. (1986). Incontinence after prostatectomy. In *The Prostate* (J. P. Blandy and B. Lytton, eds) pp. 71–81. London: Butterworth.

Kemp, E. D. (1992). Prostate cancer. *Postgraduate Medicine*, **92**, 67–89.

Killman, P. R., Milan, R. J., Boland, J. P. et al. (1987). Group treatment of secondary erectile dysfunction. *Journal of Sex and Marital Therapy*, **13**, 168–82.

Klein, J. F., Berry, C. C. and Felice, M. E. (1990). The development of a testicular self-examination instructional booklet for adolescents. *Journal of Adolescent Health Care*, **11**, 235–9.

Kockott, G., Feil, W., Ferstl, R. et al. (1980). Psychophysiological aspects of male sexual inadequacy: results of an experimental study. *Archives of Sexual Behavior*, **9**, 477–93.

Levenson, H., Olkin, R., Herzoff, N. et al. (1986). MMPI evaluation of erectile dysfunction: failure of organic versus psychogenic decision rules. *Journal of Clinical Psychology*, **42**, 752–4.

Ley, P. (1988). *Communicating With Patients: Improving Communication, Satisfaction and Compliance*. London: Croom Helm.

Lynch, T. H., Waymont, B., Beacock, B. J. M. et al. (1991). Follow up after transurethral resection of the prostate: who needs it? *British Medical Journal*, **302**, 27.

Masters, W. H. and Johnson, V. E. (1970). *Human Sexual Inadequacy*. Boston: Little Brown.

Meisler, A. W. and Carey, M. P. (1990). A critical re-evaluation of nocturnal penile tumescence monitoring in the diagnosis of erectile dysfunction. *Journal of Nervous and Mental Disorders*, **178**, 78–89.

Melman, A., Tiefer, L. and Pederson, R. (1988). Evaluation of first 406 patients in urology department based Center for Male Sexual Dysfunction. *Urology*, **32**, 6–10.

Moore, M. J., O'Sullivan, B. and Tannock, I. F. (1988). How expert physicians would wish to be treated if they had genitourinary cancer. *Journal of Clinical Oncology*, **6**, 1736–45.

Moorey, S. (1991). Adjuvant psychological therapy for anxiety and depression. In *Cancer Patient Care: Psychosocial Treatment Methods* (M. Watson, ed.) pp. 94–100. Leicester: The British Psychological Society.

Moorey, S. and Greer, S. (eds) (1989). *Psychological Therapy for Patients with Cancer: A New Approach*. London: Heinemann Medical Books.

Moul, J. W., Paulson, D. F., Dodge, R. K. et al. (1990). Delay in diagnosis and survival in testicular cancer: impact of effective therapy and changes during 18 years. *The Journal of Urology*, **143**, 520–23.

Moynihan, C. (1991). Testicular cancer. In *Cancer Patient Care: Psychosocial Treatment Methods* (M. Watson, ed.) pp. 238–59. Leicester: The British Psychological Society.

Murphy, W. G. and Brubaker, R. G. (1990). Effects of a brief theory-based intervention on the practice of testicular self-examination by high school students. *Journal of School Health*, **60**, 459–62.

Newman, H. F., Reiss, H. and Northup, J. D. (1982). Physical basis of emission, ejaculation and orgasm in the male. *Urology*, **19**, 341–50.

Parmar, H., Edwards, L., Phillips, R. H. et al. (1987). Orchidectomy vs long-acting D-Trp-6-LHRH in advanced prostatic cancer. *British Journal of Urology*, **59**, 248–54.

Parmar, H., Phillips, R. H., Edwards, L. et al. (1988). Treatment of prostatic cancer (letter). *British Medical Journal*, **296**, 1001–2.

Parmar, H., Phillips, R. H., Lightman, S. L. et al. (1985). Randomised controlled study of orchidectomy vs long-acting D-Trp-6-LHRH microcapsules in advanced prostatic carcinoma. *Lancet*, **ii**, 1201–5.

Pedersen, K. V., Carlsson, P., Varenhorst, E. et al. (1990). Screening for carcinoma of the prostate by digital rectal examination in a randomly selected population. *British Medical Journal*, **300**, 1041–4.

Post, G. J. and Belis, J. A. (1980). Delayed presentation of testicular tumors. *Southern Medical Journal*, **73**, 33.

Rieker, P. P., Edbril, S. D. and Garnick, M. B. (1985). Curative testis cancer therapy: psychosocial sequelae. *Journal of Clinical Oncology*, **3**, (8), 1117–26.

Rieker, P. P., Fitzgerald, E. M., Kalish, L. A. et al. (1989). Psychosocial factors, curative therapies and behavioral outcomes. *Cancer*, **64**, 2399–407.

Rowland, D. L. and Heiman, J. R. (1991). Self-reported and genital arousal changes in sexually dysfunctional men following a sex therapy programme. *Journal of Psychosomatic Research*, **35**, 609–19.

Sakheim, D. K., Barlow, D. H., Beck, J. G. et al. (1984). Effect of an increased awareness of erectile cues on sexual arousal. *Behavior Research and Therapy*, **22**, 151–8.

Schover, L. R., Gonzales, M. and von Eschenbach, A. C. (1986). Sexual and marital relationships after radiotherapy for seminoma. *Urology*, **28**, 2, 117–23.

Schover, L. and von Eschenbach, A. (1985). Sexual and marital relationships after treatment for nonseminomatous testicular cancer. *Urology*, **25**, 251–5.

Segraves, K. A., Segraves, R. T. and Schoenberg, H. W. (1987). Use of sexual history to differentiate organic from psychogenic impotence. *Archives of Sexual Behavior*, **16**, 125–37.

Segraves, R. T., Schoenberg, H. W., Zairns, C. K. et al. (1981). Discrimination of organic versus psychological impotence with the DSFI: a failure to replicate. *Journal of Sex and Marital Therapy*, **7**, 230–38.

Sheley, J. P., Kinchen, E. W., Morgan, D. H. et al. (1991). Limited impact of testicular self-examination promotion. *Journal of Community Health*, **16**, 117–24.

Singer, P. A., Tasch, E. S., Stocking, C. et al. (1991). Sex or survival: trade-offs between quality and quantity of life. *Journal of Clinical Oncology*, **9**, 328–34.

Slag, M. F., Morley, J. E., Elson, M. K. et al. (1983). Impotence in medical clinic outpatients. *Journal of the American Medical Association*, **249**, 1736–40.

Speckens, A. E. M., Hengeveld, M. W., Lycklama a Nijeholt, G. A. B. et al. (1993). Discrimination between psychogenic and organic erectile dysfunction. *Journal of Psychosomatic Research*, **37**, 135–45.

Spector, K. R. and Boyle, M. (1986). The prevalence and perceived aetiology of male sexual problems in a non-clinical sample. *British Journal of Medical Psychology*, **59**, 351–8.

Tross, S. (1989). Psychological adjustment in testicular cancer. In *Handbook of Psycho-oncology: Psychological Care of the Patient With Cancer* (J. C. Holland and J. H. Rowland, eds) pp. 240–45. New York: Oxford University Press.

Vogt, H. B. and McHale, M. S. (1992). Testicular cancer: role of primary care physicians in screening and education. *Postgraduate Medicine*, **92**, 93–101.

Williams, C. J. (1990). *Cancer Biology and Management: An Introduction*. Chichester: John Wiley and Sons.

Zohar, J., Meiraz, D., Maoz, B. et al. (1976). Factors influencing sexual activity after prostatectomy: a prospective study. *Journal of Urology*, **116**, 332–4.

# 7

# Family planning and reproductive decisions[1]

Elphis Christopher

Fertility control is not a modern phenomenon. As long as people have been aware of their capacity to reproduce they have attempted to control the number of children they have, when they have them and often particular characteristics of their children, especially gender. In the twentieth century we are technically able to do all of these things more reliably than at any other time in the past. However, despite 1960s jubilation about 'the pill' as the ultimate key to sex without conception, unwanted pregnancies still occur, even in wealthy urbanized western societies. In this chapter, Elphis Christopher uses her experience as a family planning doctor in North London over twenty-five years to explore the many and varied factors which have been found in clinic work to influence contraceptive use. The case studies and descriptions of family planning services in this chapter clearly demonstrate the complexity of contraceptive choice and use, and place it in its sociocultural and developmental context. Is everyone concerned about contraception? Which factors are important? What are the roles of family, culture, education, religion, individual identity, sexuality, and contraceptive availability?

## Introduction

This paper will look at factors involved in both the use of contraception and reproductive decision making. Knowledge about these factors has been gained through over twenty years' experience in providing contraceptive/family planning advice in a variety of settings in a North London borough (Haringey). The settings have been an ordinary family planning clinic since 1966, a young people's clinic and domiciliary family planning (that is home visiting to give women/couples family planning advice) both since 1968. The work of the latter has been previously documented (Christopher, Kellaher and Von Koch, 1980). Case studies will be used to illustrate the texts.

## Background

Haringey has a population of around 200 000 which is multiethnic in origin, largely Afro-Caribbean, Asian (latterly Bangladeshi), Cypriot and Irish. The population is young compared with that of England and Wales: 47 per cent is made up of people between the ages of 15 and 44.

The number of births have been around 3300 for the last seventeen years with an increasing number outside marriage (1288 in 1987, 37 per cent). This compares to 27 per cent nationally. The crude live birth rate (live births per 1000 resident population) is 17.4 compared to 13.6 for England and Wales. The

[1] This paper first appeared in the *Journal of Reproductive and Infant Psychology* (1991) **9**: 217–26.

**Table 7.1** Ages of those having
abortions in Haringey in 1989

| | |
|---|---|
| Under 16 | 13 |
| 16–19 | 241 |
| 20–24 | 825 |
| 25–34 | 890 |
| 35–44 | 184 |
| 45+ | 2 |

general fertility rate (the number of live births per 1000 women aged 15–44) is 73.2 for Haringey compared to 63 for England.

Abortion has been made readily available since 1973 with a day care service through the National Health Service at the local hospital (North Middlesex). However only half the terminations performed on Haringey women are done through the National Health Service.

The actual number of abortions has been rising steadily with Haringey having the highest number in the North East Thames Region. In 1989 there was a total of 2155 terminations performed, with 1619 (75 per cent) carried out on single (never married) women and 367 (17 per cent) on married women, 169 to widowed, separated, divorced and not known categories. Ages of the women and number of previous pregnancies are shown in Tables 7.1 and 7.2.

**Table 7.2** Parity of those having abortions
in Haringey in 1989

| | |
|---|---|
| No previous pregnancies | 1328 |
| 1–3 pregnancies | 751 |
| 4+ | 76 |

## Family planning services provided

There are twenty-three family planning clinic sessions per week. They are situated around the borough mainly, running in the evenings, offering all methods of contraception including emergency or post coital contraception. The majority of general practitioners also offer a contraceptive service though the emphasis is on the oral contraceptive pill.

**Table 7.3** The ethnic origin of the women referred to the
domiciliary family planning service

| | |
|---|---|
| English, Scot, Welsh | 1091 (36%) |
| Eire | 231 (7%) |
| Caribbean | 1158 (38%) |
| Cypriot (Greek & Turkish) | 178 (6%) |
| Asian (from India, Pakistan, Bangladesh) | 393 (13%) |
| + Others | |

The domiciliary family planning service run by a doctor and three nurses working part-time has visited 3051 women during the years 1968–89. There are around 100–120 referrals to the service with one-third self-referred and the rest being referred by professionals, mainly health visitors.

Of these 3051, 47 per cent (1435) were single, never married women while 45 per cent (1379) were married with 8 per cent (237) separated or divorced. Ethnic origin is shown in Table 7.3.

## The 'factors wheel'

It might be helpful to look at the factors involved in reproductive decision making in the form of a wheel, Figure 7.1.

Although divided into eight equal segments the different factors are not compartmentalized but are often overlapping and interlocking. Some factors are obviously more important than others for individuals, couples and societies and will vary over time, changing with increasing knowledge and experience both about contraception and abortion and the reality of pregnancy, child rearing and population pressures. Altered socio-economic circumstances and changing relationships (separation, divorce) will also have differing consequences for reproductive decision making. Running like a leitmotif through all the aspects of

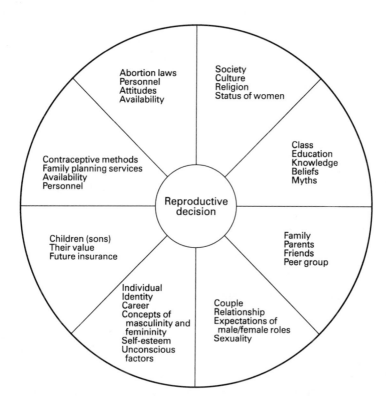

**Figure 7.1** Family planning 'factors wheel'

family planning is the status of women and how their role is perceived; whether they are seen principally as child-bearers. Attitudes towards sexuality and its expression – whether regarded mainly for procreation or pleasure – can have profound consequences for reproductive decision making. Sexual activity is often impulsive and unplanned for, tied up as it is with powerful and often overwhelming desires and emotions, whereas the use of contraception requires forethought and conscious effort. At some level most couples would prefer *not* to be bothered about contraception.

## Society, culture and religion

Societal attitudes towards reproduction, fertility, sexuality and family planning are important in so far as they create the general climate in which the decisions about whether to have children, how many and whether to use contraception exist. Thus there is the acceptance/non-acceptance of the very idea or concept of planning, spacing or limiting family size. This in turn will influence whether services are provided to facilitate reproductive choices. All religions are pronatalist and anti-abortion. Some may allow a pregnancy to be terminated for specific reasons, for instance where the woman's life is at risk. Religions may not be adverse to planning or limiting one's family but may be divided as to the means to do it, e.g. abstinence or natural family planning for Roman Catholics. Among Orthodox Jews the *man* must not impede the sperm hence male methods are not used though the women may use contraception. For Moslems both the husband and wife must agree to the use of birth control and abortion may be allowed to prevent a handicapped child. The genitals can only be touched with the left hand (making diaphragm usage difficult). Women may not go to the mosque when menstruating and they can only be examined by female doctors. Among Hindus, sons are important to enable certain rituals to be performed for the father when he dies. Daughters are a liability as they require the provision of dowries.

Cultural factors rather than religious ones appear more significant among Caribbean women. Birth outside marriage is not considered a social stigma (in some Caribbean islands 80 per cent of births are outside marriage). Fertility (or the proof of it) is considered very important. A barren woman is likened to a mule. Attitudes to abortion are negative (though abortion is often requested) summed up in the phrase 'her womb is a graveyard'.

How seriously people take their religion and their perception and knowledge of what it actually says with regard to family planning obviously varies. Thus in giving contraceptive advice it is essential to ascertain the person's views and to avoid making assumptions about their beliefs and attitudes.

## Class, education and knowledge

Generally speaking those in long-term education and from a higher socio-economic class tend to have smaller families regardless of cultural/societal/religious influences, summed up by the words of a popular song 'the rich get rich and the poor get children'. However, there are exceptions to this, possibly related to aspirations, expectations and economic success. In the 1930s in Britain 'the poor' did reduce family size, women relying heavily (and at high cost to their health) on backstreet abortion. Indeed, the efforts to change the abortion law in this country were spurred on by the high maternal mortality as a result of back street abortion in the 1930s.

In developing countries where many present day immigrant families originate, 'the poor' do tend to have many children. This is because of the high infant mortality (1 in 10 births in some places), the need for sons and children being seen as a source of help and wealth: hands for the field and insurance for old age. In Britain today some large families (five and more children) are to be found both among the well off and the poor.

In 1985, social classes I and II making up 25 per cent of the population accounted for 30 per cent of all births. IV and V, making up 20 per cent of the population, accounted for 19 per cent of births, although births outside marriage largely belonged to social classes IV and V (OPCS, 1985).

Included in education and knowledge is the information about sex and contraception. Although sex education is now included as part of the core curriculum together with health education, there is still controversy about the 'who', 'what', 'how much' and 'when' aspects of providing it. For years there has been a current belief that teaching teenagers about contraception will be giving them a licence to have sex. Sexual ignorance is seen as bliss. The teenager is often caught in a double bind. There is a loss of face for an adolescent to admit to ignorance on sexual matters though he or she may desperately need help. There is considerable anxiety about sex education and its effects among certain ethnic groups in Britain, particularly Cypriot and Asian. There is a fear of girls losing their 'respect', i.e. their virginity, if they are taught about sex. Myths come into play with ignorance about the body and how it functions: female genitalia are seen as 'one hole down below'; things 'get lost inside'; only mutual orgasms can get you pregnant; 'you can't get pregnant if he pulls out'; nor can you if you jump up and down after sex or 'pee' (thereby hoping to flush sperm out).

**Family, parents, friends and peer group**

In patriarchal cultures such as Asian and Cypriot, marriages are arranged or semi-arranged. A marriage is not considered a true one unless there are children. Children, especially sons, increase the status of the woman within those societies. There is shame if younger siblings produce children before older ones when both are married. There is pressure from parents on their children to reproduce. This can be seen in all societies. Peer group pressure is significant among certain teenage groups especially girls who have been in local authority care.

**The couple**

The stability and quality of the relationship can determine whether contraception is used and which partner uses it. Where there is trust and openness in the relationship, contraception can be accepted more readily though there may be resentment that it is needed and a dislike of the actual methods. An unintended pregnancy is more likely to occur when the relationship is unstable, beginning or ending, as there may be no, or erratic, use of contraception. Education and counselling to promote good relationships may be as important as contraceptive counselling regarding the methods themselves (Skinner, 1989). The sexual relationship may be for mutual pleasure and joy or it may be to control, dominate or compensate for feelings of inadequacy. The relationship may be to the genitals rather than the whole person, collecting vaginas in the manner of collecting scalps. Allowing a pregnancy 'to happen' can be a way of testing the relationship, holding on to the partner. One partner only may want a pregnancy; methods may then be sabotaged. Pregnancy can be used to control the woman especially where there is violence in a relationship. There may be stereotyped role expectations of being male and female. Thus to be female must mean being a mother. Couples can make a deliberate conscious choice to have a child with delight in children and rearing them with a reasonably realistic appraisal of what is required. However, many if not most pregnancies are 'accidental', sometimes welcome, sometimes not. The reproductive decision whether to continue with the pregnancy may then depend on the availability of abortion. The pregnancy itself needs to be defined. A pregnancy may be unplanned, unintended but wanted. It may be planned and intended but later as circumstances change become unwanted. The pregnancy may be unplanned but wanted though again the woman may seek termination if the difficulties of having the child are too great.

Sexual problems can influence the reproductive decision. The couple may think the use of contraception is pointless if the man experiences premature ejaculation or the woman loses her sexual desire or if there is infrequent sex. Indeed, such problems can surface as a result of a consultation about contraception. The contraceptive methods themselves may cause sexual problems, e.g. a man may lose his erection with the condom. This may influence against the use of contraception. Sexual problems can be a cause of infertility, for example where the relationship has not been consummated or where the man has delayed or retarded ejaculation. The experience of infertility, its investigation and treatment can in turn cause sexual difficulties.

## The individual

The reproductive decision can be tied to identity issues and how far the individual's identity as a man or woman is bound up with the ability to have children. Masculinity and femininity can be equated with virility and fertility. There may be anxiety about not being able to have a child. This is particularly pertinent with regard to teenagers with low self-esteem. Having a baby is the one 'good' thing they can achieve. For the man who feels inadequate and unable to compete with other men, getting a woman pregnant may satisfy a need to 'prove' himself: he really is a man. Feelings about sex and one's own sexuality can determine whether contraception is used. Is sex solely for procreation? Is sex made acceptable by allowing conception or the possibility of it? Is sex for pleasure regarded as disgusting, shameful and dirty? The person can own and take charge of his or her own sexuality or simply leave things to chance – deciding by not deciding.

For women, especially 'career women', there is the pressure of the biological time clock which can cause great conflict and confusion about a possible pregnancy. There can be the savage irony of having spent years diligently using contraception to avoid pregnancy only to discover that one is infertile. There is the experience of fertility, childbirth and children which itself influences and determines future reproductive decisions. For example, bad birth experiences can change attitudes both with regard to future pregnancies and the use of contraception. Guilt about a pregnancy that was terminated can lead to taking chances with contraception to make some kind of reparation.

There are also unconscious factors at work. The 'need' for a baby can be confused with the wish to be thought of as normal. The baby can represent something 'good' being produced from 'bad' sex or a 'bad body' or 'bad relationship'. The baby can be a replacement for loss of any kind. Being pregnant – literally being filled with new life – can compensate for inner feelings of emptiness. Once delivered of the baby, the woman may be anxious to get pregnant soon afterwards and resent discussion about contraception. The baby can represent one's own baby self to be loved vicariously. Pregnancy and children can enhance status. Mothers, although not necessarily treated well, are regarded as 'good'. There may be rivalry with or envy of one's own mother or a sibling to be a better mother or a bid to outdo them, i.e. have more children. Pregnancy or the pregnant state may be feared, the fetus seen as a parasite devouring and invading the woman's body. A split between mind and body can occur with the adult body which can get pregnant and the mind or feelings which do not feel grown up enough or ready to envisage getting pregnant. In these situations there can be the sense of the body betraying the person, exemplified by the following expressions when pregnancy is diagnosed: 'I don't believe it', 'It can't be', 'I didn't think it would happen to me.'

Fatalistic attitudes can affect the use of contraception. Where things just happen and life events feel uncontrollable then there may be feelings that fertility cannot be controlled. Indeed, the very effectiveness of some methods of contraception may so threaten and challenge these attitudes that the method may be sabotaged. As one women put it: 'If you're meant to have a lot of children then even that pill can't stop you.'

## Children

A baby or a child represents a new beginning, new hope. The child may be expected to live the life its parents wanted to live. Children confer adult status, carry on the family name, are an insurance for old age, keep you young, ensure some kind of immortality, keep the marriage and relationship together, prevent boredom, loneliness, provide interest, entertainment, satisfy the need to be needed, define a role in life and provide stability. They can be used as a bastion against the world by creating one's own tribe. Children can be seen as a nuisance, too demanding, too threatening, too unpredictable, testing the maturity of the individual or couple. There may be an obsession with getting a son or daughter.

## Contraception and family planning

It is a truism that has now become a cliche that the perfect or ideal method of contraception does not exist. The ideal method would be 100 per cent effective as a contraceptive, instantly reversible, not interfere with the sex act and have no side-effects. It should also be a method in which the 'default state' is contraception with the need for an easy positive action by the user in order to achieve a conception, e.g. a completely side-effect-free and 100 per cent effective intrauterine device which the user could either leave alone or remove herself when she wanted to conceive. The method which individuals choose is usually one that they can cope with in terms of risks and benefits and may change with experience and the need for greater effectiveness. It is a present day irony that the *perceived risks* are greater, for example, than the actual risks of taking the oral contraceptive pill. This obviously affects people's attitudes to the methods. Thus frequent comments heard during contraceptive consultations are:

- the pill kills
- the coil makes you sterile or damages the baby
- like putting your whatsit (penis) in a bed of thorns (the threads of the intra-uterine device)
- the cap is too messy; by the time you've put it in you've gone off the boil
- the government puts a hole in every tenth condom to keep the population up
  the condom is a passion-killer
  you need skin to skin for good sex
  using a condom is like going to bed in your wellingtons or having a bath with your socks on
  allergic to them rubbers (losing the erection)
- the injectable contraceptives make you sterile, give you cancer, make you hairy, put you off sex.

Thus erratic or non-use of contraception can be due to a dislike/fear of the methods, resentment at having to use a method or being the one expected to take precautions, especially for those who do not enjoy sex. If there is envy of the other's sexual enjoyment, not using contraception can be used as a way of trying to control or limit it. If there is guilt or conflict about sexual desires or activity (especially where the woman has a history of sexual abuse) then contraception may not be used. If there is a difficulty in owning one's sexuality and taking responsibility for it, there may be a reluctance to use contraception:

'thought she was on the pill'
'thought he was being careful'
'didn't know him well enough to take the pill'
'didn't need anything because not doing nothing'
'mothers are the ones who get pregnant, not me'

Contraceptive services and the attitudes of the personnel providing them can affect the reproductive decision. Services need to be easily accessible and held at convenient times. Staff need to be welcoming, non-judgemental and sensitive, especially to the person's need for privacy, confidentiality and unbiased information and advice together with careful teaching about the method. A woman doctor may be essential, for example, for certain Moslem women who will not see a male doctor about such intimate matters. Negative or brusque unsympathetic attitudes on the part of family planning staff can lead to non-use of a method or poor compliance.

**Abortion and abortion services**

Over 180 000 women chose to abort their pregnancies in 1989 in England and Wales. The ratio of abortions to live births is one to three/four live births. More than one woman in three experiencing the present fertility rates in her lifetime might have a legal abortion in England and Wales (Clarke, 1988). Although there are a large number of terminations carried out every year and the number has risen steadily since the Abortion Act was passed in 1986, Britain actually has one of the lowest rates of abortion per woman lifetime compared to other European countries where there is legalized abortion. It is evident that women, especially those single women in their 20s with no or one child (proportionately the highest number of those having terminations), are availing themselves of the option to abort a pregnancy rather than have an unwanted child.

The reproductive decision can be affected by the availability of an abortion service and by the attitudes of the medical and nursing staff caring for the woman. If women are made to feel more guilty than they already do and have not been allowed to grieve properly, there may be another pregnancy within a short time. Few studies looking at the psychological sequelae actually address this (Christopher, 1987).

# Some case studies

## Society, culture and religion

### Case 1

A Bangladeshi Moslem woman of 42 years with eleven children was visited at home by the linkworker and domiciliary family planning doctor. She and her husband decided she should take the oral progestogen-only pill. She took it for a year without problems then on one visit the husband who appeared to have been hiding in the bushes outside the house rushed in shouting, 'No pills, no pills'. His wife looked bewildered. It was later learnt from the health visitor that she had had a twelfth child. The woman's views about this were not discovered.

Many of the women visited in the early years of the domiciliary family planning service had large families with six or more children. This included women of a variety of ethnic and religious backgrounds. Many of these women requested sterilization as they wanted no more children. The local gynaecologist who was a member of the Plymouth Brethren sect, refused either to do terminations or sterilizations. The women had to be referred to hospitals outside the area. Interestingly, few of their daughters have gone on to have such large families even though some, especially those of Caribbean origin, have had their first child in early or mid teens. Support through the domiciliary family planning service has enabled these girls to exercise greater control over their fertility.

The actual experience of having and rearing children can counter societal/religious views and beliefs.

### Case 2

Mrs E. was 23 years when first visited, a strict Jehovah's Witness with two children aged 2 years and 1 year. She was adamant that she wanted no foreign chemicals and wished to rely on 'natural family planning'. She was taught how to predict ovulation (thermo-symptal and mucus method). The method worked for a year then she became pregnant again. She could not contemplate an abortion so she had the child, a boy, which is what she wanted. After this pregnancy, she decided to take no more chances. She opted for the oral contraceptive pill which she has taken for 6 years without problems.

## Conflict in the relationship

### Case 3

Mrs K., 32 years old with six children, found fault with every method. She would try a method and then delight in telling the domiciliary doctor that it was no use. Eventually having defeated all the methods (and the doctor!) she said 'He' meaning her husband, 'would have to be done' (vasectomy). Mr K. sat quiet and defeated. It was hard to believe he was the demon that Mrs K. described. He used to drink heavily and become aggressive. When sober he was henpecked. He agreed to have the vasectomy. He failed to keep two appointments and despite Mrs K. refusing contraception and at the same time saying she wanted no further pregnancies she became pregnant. It seemed a case of 'cutting off one's nose to spite one's face!' Mrs K. was furious with Mr K. and the doctor for the pregnancy happening. The delivery proved difficult; a breech birth. Mrs K. decided she had had enough and opted for the oral contraceptive pill which she took without any problems. She subsequently referred several of her daughters to the domiciliary family planning service.

### Unconscious conflict about family planning versus motherhood

*Case 4*

Miss L. was 21 years old and had had four children in as many years. She was a loving mother but perpetually exhausted. She seemed set to follow her mother's pattern of fourteen children. Several of these children, including herself, had been in the care of the local authority from time to time. It became increasingly evident with each meeting that a tremendous struggle was going on inside of Miss L. as shown by her complaints about contraception and her feelings towards the doctor which were sometimes hostile and at others welcoming. On the latter occasions she would express great interest and curiosity in family planning work. The doctor alternatively felt like a warm supportive mother and a hater of babies – someone out to prevent her and all the other women being visited through the domiciliary family planning service from having all the babies she and they longed to have. At one visit Miss L. yet again voiced her anxiety about the possible harm the coil was doing to her 'insides'. The doctor decided to tell Miss L. about the way she made her feel and wondered if this reflected the way she (Miss L.) was feeling. Miss L. then began to talk about her mother who had made her feel that having babies was the normal thing to do and that they should not be prevented. She also knew that her mother had great difficulty in actually caring for her children. Admitting this made Miss L. feel guilty about her mother. The doctor commented that she did not have to be either like or unlike her mother: she could be herself. It was obvious that she loved her children but knew she did not have endless patience or energy and what could be managed with four children could not be managed with fourteen. This seemed to free her in some way as there were no further complaints about her coil. Her youngest child is now 11 years old.

## Summary

The factors involved in reproductive decision making are diverse and complex. Which ones are the most significant can vary from person to person and over time and can change with the actual experience of being pregnant and having children. Thus the giving of contraceptive advice while seemingly simple in some of its aspects (for example in the provision of easily accessible and free services and methods) can also be exceedingly complex, involving as it does the most private and intimate areas of an individual or couple's life.

# Applications

### 1. Be aware of the decision making process
The decision to use or not to use contraception is a complex one and is influenced by many factors. Practitioners need to be aware that whilst for some people the decision is straightforward, for others it is more difficult. This group may need more time to think and talk about their decision.

### 2. Counselling or advice?
The use of contraception may touch on many areas of life – sexuality, relationships, self-identity, ideas about gender, career aspirations, and so on. The practitioner may need to be a counsellor as well as an advisor.

### 3. Be sensitive and flexible
There are few strict rules about the choice of contraceptive technique. Practitioners need to be sensitive to the individual needs of their clients and flexible in the advice given.

## Further reading

Christopher, E. (1987). *Sexuality and Birth Control in Community Work*. 2nd edn, London and New York: Tavistock Publications.

Montford, H. and Skrine, R. (1993). *Contraceptive Care*. London and New York: Chapman and Hall.

Walker, A. and McNeill, E. (eds) (1991). Family Planning and Reproductive Decisions: Theme Issues of the *Journal of Reproductive and Infant Psychology*, **9**, 4, 215–69.

## References

Christopher, E. (1987). *Sexuality and Birth Control in Community Work*. 2nd edn, London and New York: Tavistock Publications.

Christopher, E., Kellaher, L., Von Koch, A. (1980). A survey of 1300 women referred to the Haringey Domiciliary Family Planning Service 1968–1975. Research Report No. 3. Survey Research Unit, Department of Applied Social Studies, The Polytechnic of North London.

Clarke, M. (1988). Fertility and legal abortion in England and Wales: performance indicators for family planning services. *British Medical Journal*, **297**, 832–3.

OPCS (1985). Social Class Series FM/No. 11.

Skinner, C. (1989). *The Elusive Mr Right*. London: Carolina Publications.

# 8

# Premarital contraceptive use[1]

## Paschal Sheeran, David White and Keith Phillips

In the previous chapter, family planning was shown to be a complex and multi-faceted process. The factors which influence the decision to contracept, and the choice of contraception vary at different life stages and are strongly influenced by culture and other social factors. In this chapter, Paschal Sheeran, David White and Keith Phillips consider the psychosocial factors which influence contraceptive use at one particular life stage – that is among young people who have not yet made a long-term commitment to a relationship. This group is of particular interest because of the rate of adolescent pregnancy and more recently because of the risk of HIV infection. This chapter reviews the psychological theories which have been used to explain contraceptive use in this group. Is contraceptive use part of a decision-making process? Are attitudes to different types of contraception important? Are there any differences between those young people who use contraception and those who do not? Are psychological theories enough to explain contraceptive behaviour?

## Introduction

Despite the availability of effective contraceptive technology large numbers of young people in western countries continue to experience unwanted pregnancy (Alan Guttmacher Institute, 1981; Jones, Forrest, Goldman et al., 1985). Those factors which enable or hinder effective contraceptive use (CU) by people who do not actively want to become pregnant have been the subject of a great deal of research by social scientists. This paper reviews psychological literature in this area outlining the major theoretical frameworks used in research and summarizing findings with respect to the types of variables significantly associated with CU. It should be noted that this literature is explicitly concerned with the issue of *pregnancy avoidance* and has not, at least as yet, examined CU as it pertains to the prevention of sexually transmitted diseases such as HIV/AIDS.

While culture is clearly a central factor in contraceptive behaviour (e.g. Mauldin and Segal, 1988) the influence of this variable lies beyond the scope of the present work. Consequently, the findings reported here are most applicable to western countries. Only studies published since 1970 are included since changes in sexual standards limit the generalizability of previous research (Chilman, 1983) and since studies conducted in previous decades are primarily descriptive (Morrison, 1985).

A majority of psychological studies of CU use second- or third-level student samples while the remainder usually employ attenders at abortion or family planning (FP) clinics. Because studies frequently do not provide precise information on respondents' marital status, social class, age or ethnicity or

[1] This paper first appeared in the *Journal of Reproductive and Infant Psychology* (1991) **9**: 253–69. Copyright © 1991 by Society for Reproductive and Infant Psychology. Reprinted with permission.

clearly indicate the response rate obtained, whether the research was anonymous and/or confidential or whether payment in the form of money or course credit was used to motivate respondents, it is difficult to characterize extant research in terms of these variables. A majority of studies, however, appear to have sampled never-married individuals between the ages of 13 and 25 years. Respondents were usually white and middle class with a small number of exceptions (e.g. Jones and Phillibur, 1983). Cross-sectional questionnaire designs were used by the vast majority of researchers while structured interviews were used in the remaining studies. Relatively few longitudinal or experimental studies have been conducted in this area. Studies using samples of females-only outnumber mixed-sex samples by about two to one. This may reflect the fact that most contraceptive methods are used only by women or that females are a more accessible population for research in this area (Beck and Davies, 1982). Unfortunately, Finkel and Finkel's (1983) charge that males are 'the forgotten partner' in research on CU continues to be the case. Similarly, there appears to be no research which has examined birth control from a *joint* decision-making perspective.

A major difficulty associated with reviewing the literature in this area is the wide variety of operationalizations of CU (see Herold, 1981a). Studies have examined whether or not contraception was used during first intercourse, last intercourse or with respondents' last 'serious' or 'casual' partner. Similarly, the consistency with which contraception has been used over specific time periods and the effectiveness of the method used have been studied both separately and in a combined index where frequent use of an unreliable method is roughly equated with infrequent use of a reliable method.

Morrison (1985) points out that the variety of classifications of contraceptive methods made by researchers is problematic since characteristics of contraceptive methods are confounded. Different researchers may group contraceptive methods differently. For example, birth control pills have been classified as a 'reliable method' with condoms, as a 'female-controlled method' with foam, as a 'coitus-independent method' with the rhythm method or as a 'prescription-based method' with the intrauterine device (IUD). Moreover, researchers may simply disagree on which methods should be included in 'effective' vs 'ineffective' categories (see, e.g. Fox, 1977 vs Thompson and Spanier, 1978 vs Foreit and Foreit, 1981). Operationalizations of CU in terms of compliance with a regimen prescribed by a FP clinic suffer from the difficulties that only those who intend to use contraception to begin with are included in the study while not returning for a clinic appointment may be due to a variety of reasons other than the one that is generally assumed, namely that contraception has been discontinued. Similarly, unintended pregnancy is a poor measure of contraceptive non-use since pregnancy may be due to contraceptive failure rather than non-use (Oskamp and Mindick, 1983).

Perhaps the most serious problem with research in this area is its piecemeal nature. Milan and Kilmann (1987) point out that few studies have used measures which incorporate the results of previous research. The multiplicity of operationalizations of CU is paralleled by a wide variety of operationalizations of predictor variables. Many studies examine associations between CU and small numbers of variables selected without apparent reference to particular theoretical models. Studies which explicitly test conceptual accounts are relatively rare. Based on these considerations, this review first outlines the theoretical accounts of CU which have been proposed and examines the empirical evidence supporting these models. Secondly, a synthesis of research findings is presented. This section of the review is organized around the types of factors which have been shown to be significantly related to CU. These factors can broadly be distinguished in terms of their intrapersonal vs interpersonal emphases. Five factors are considered: background factors; knowledge, attitudes and beliefs; interpersonal factors; personality factors and situational influences.

## Theoretical accounts of contraceptive use

Three criteria were used to judge whether a particular theory should be included in the present review. First, the theory must be explicitly concerned with CU in the sense of pregnancy avoidance rather than prevention of sexually transmitted disease such as HIV/AIDS. Second, the theory should make a substantive multivariate contribution to research in this area and possess some conceptual distinctiveness. And third, the framework should propose a causal or developmental priority of certain variables over others and/or indicate the presence of direct vs indirect effects. On this basis nine accounts were included. These theories can usefully be distinguished in terms of their *decision-making* vs *developmental* perspectives. Table 8.1 summarizes the theories and their major conceptual contributions.

### Decision models

Decision models are derived from subjective expected utility (SEU) theory (Edwards, 1954) and have received considerable attention in the psychological literature. SEU theory suggests that people make subjective estimates of the probability that costs and benefits will result from particular courses of action and that they then choose that course which gives greatest benefit and least cost in material, social and psychological terms. Thus Luker's (1975) account which uses SEU theory in the specific context of CU suggests that people weigh the probability of pregnancy and its costs and benefits against the costs and benefits of contraception in making their decision about birth control. Luker's singular contribution is her undermining of the often made assumptions that contraception has no costs for women or that pregnancy has no benefits. Luker's theory is unique in that the probability of reversing pregnancy (e.g. through abortion) is specifically included in her formulation. She also acknowledges a variety of social and psychological pressure to become pregnant under a category of 'interpersonal exigencies'. Foreit and Foreit's (1981) empirical test of Luker's theory, however, found little support for the model. Associations between CU and perceived pregnancy risk, benefits of pregnancy and willingness to seek abortion were not statistically reliable. Foreit and Foreit's operationalizations of these variables are, arguably, rather poor, however. Moreover, these researchers did not operationalize either the costs/benefits of contraception or interpersonal exigencies. Although not empirically supported, Luker's remains a popular theory.

Fishbein's theory of reasoned action (Fishbein, 1972; Fishbein and Ajzen, 1975) extends SEU theory to encompass both social influence and intention

**Table 8.1** Summary of major theoretical accounts of contraceptive use

| Account | Major concepts | Empirical studies |
|---|---|---|
| *Decision theories* | | |
| Luker (1975) | Cost of contraception; benefits of pregnancy; subjective probability assigned to pregnancy; probability of reversing pregnancy; interpersonal exigencies | Foreit and Foreit, 1981 |
| Fishbein (1972) | Behavioural intention; attitude towards contraception; subjective norm | Fishbein and Jaccard, 1973; Jaccard and Davisdson, 1972; Jorgensen and Sonstegard, 1984; Cohen, Severy and Ahtola, 1978; Ewald and Roberts, 1981; Werner and Middlestadt, 1979 |
| Byrne, Jazwinski, DeNinno and Fisher (1977), Byrne (1983) | Emotional responses (to sex); sexual attitudes; information; expectations about pregnancy and contraception; norms; level of arousal | Fisher, 1984; Fisher, Bryne, Edmunds et al., 1979 |
| Reiss, Banwart and Foreman (1975) | Endorsement of sexual choices; self-assurance; early information on sex and contraception; attitude-behaviour congruence; dyadic commitment | Reiss, Banwart and Foreman, 1975; DeLamater and MacCorquodale, 1978 |
| Herold and McNamee (1982) | Peer/parent acceptance of premarital intercourse; guilt about intercourse; lifetime partners; frequency of intercourse; involvement with partner; partner influence; contraceptive attitude | Herold and McNamee, 1982 |
| Lowe and Radius (1987) | Susceptibility to pregnancy; seriousness of pregnancy; costs and benefits of contraceptive use | Lowe and Radius, 1987 |
| *Developmental theories* | | |
| Lindemann (1974, 1977) | Three stages ('natural', 'peer-prescription' and 'expert') characterized by increasing sexual activity and acceptance of sexuality into the self-concept | |
| Rains (1971) | 'Moral ambivalence', acceptance of contraceptive responsibility; being 'in love'; exclusive dating; longer-term sexual involvement; acknowledging sex is likely in the future | DeLamater and MacCorquodale, 1978 |
| DeLamater (1983) | Premarital sexual standards; intimacy of relationship; frequency of intercourse; perceived probability of pregnancy; cognitive assessment of pregnancy/previous contraceptive experience | |

variables. Beliefs about the consequences of CU multiplied by the individual's evaluation of those consequences form the person's *attitude towards contraception*. Beliefs about whether significant others think the person should or should not use contraception (*normative beliefs*) multiplied by one's motivation to comply with those others form the person's *subjective norm*. Individual's attitude and subjective norm additively predict their *behavioural intentions* to use contraception. These intentions are the immediate predictors of contraceptive behaviour and mediate the influence of other variables including variables extraneous to the model. Empirical tests of Fishbein's formulation are quite supportive. Jaccard and Davidson (1972), Davidson and Jaccard (1975) and Cohen, Severy and Ahtola (1978) found multiple correlations of 0.84, 0.81 and 0.48 respectively between model components and intentions to use oral contraceptives but did not measure behaviours. Werner and Middlestadt (1979) obtained a multiple correlation of 0.55 between attitudes, subjective norms and use of oral contraceptives in a study of sixty-one college females and report a zero-order correlation of 0.83 between intention and behaviour. Jorgensen and Sonstegard's (1984) test of the model with 244 female adolescents aged 13 to 18, however, explained, at most, only 11 per cent of the variance on a number of CU variables. There researchers, it should be noted, used only three items to measure attitude towards contraception and did not operationalize behavioural intention.

Byrne's Sexual Behaviour Sequence (Byrne, Jazwinski, DeNinno and Fisher, 1977; Byrne, 1983) includes most of the elements of the Fishbein model but is distinguished by its inclusion of sexual arousal, emotional responses to sex and its focus upon the information system which supports attitudinal and normative analyses (Schinke, Gilchrist and Small, 1979). While this perspective has been fully elaborated as an account of CU by Byrne (1983) it has only been partially subjected to empirical test. Research work to date has been primarily concerned with the development and validation of a measure of learned emotional responses to sexuality termed *erotophilia–erotophobia*. Erotophobic individuals show generalized avoidance responses to sexual cues since they are dispositionally predisposed to finding these cues aversive. Erotophilic individuals, on the other hand, find these cues pleasurable and show approach responses. Fisher's (1984) prospective study of ninety-six college males found correlations of 0.33 and 0.44 with condom use over a 4-week period for erotophilia–erotophobia and behavioural intention respectively. The independent measures were not significantly related ($r = -0.08$). Interestingly, multiple regression analysis showed that both erotophilia–erotophobia and intention contributed uniquely to the prediction of condom use (multiple $R = 0.57$). This finding undermines Fishbein's contention that the effects of variables extraneous to his model are mediated by behavioural intention. Erotophilia–erotophobia is considered in greater detail in the section on personality influences.

Another important account of CU which has not received a great deal of empirical attention is that of Reiss, Banwart and Foreman (1975). This model has five major components: endorsement of sexual choices (including, e.g. permissiveness, religiosity, attitude to female initiation of sexual activity); self-assurance; early information on sex and contraception; congruity between premarital sexual standards and behaviour and the extent of dyadic commitment (e.g. engaged vs 'going steady'). Unfortunately, the study did not obtain support for the third or fourth components. Similarly, DeLamater and MacCorquodale's (1978) test of the model found that only operationalizations of endorsement of sexual choices were significantly but weakly correlated with contraceptive use among women or men.

A more recent decision-making account which has been tested using path analysis is that of Herold and McNamee (1982). A total of eight variables comprise their framework. These include parental and peer norms for acceptance of premarital intercourse; number of lifetime sexual partners; guilt about intercourse and contraceptive attitudes. Three relationship variables are also operationalized: involvement with partner, partner influence to use contraception and frequency of intercourse. Herold and McNamee obtained significant direct paths for peer norms, lifetime partners, partner involvement and influence, guilt and contraceptive attitudes and the dependent variable, contraceptive method used at last intercourse. Parental norms and intercourse frequency had significant indirect effects via number of lifetime partners in the case of the former and via partner influence and guilt in the case of the latter. The total variance explained by the model was quite impressive $R^2 = 0.37$). Some caution might be appropriate in interpreting these findings, however, since all the variables were measured at a single time-point and inferences about causality require further longitudinal study.

The final decision model considered here (Lowe and Radius, 1987) draws upon a variant of SEU which has proven utility in the area of preventive health behaviour – the health belief model (HBM, Rosenstock, 1974). The major concepts associated with this framework are perceived susceptibility to pregnancy, the perceived seriousness of pregnancy and perceived barriers to, and benefits of, CU. These are the central variables in the model and are believed to mediate the effects of background variables such as age, sex and race on behaviour. Lowe and Radius' study, however, expands the HBM analysis to include personality variables (self-esteem, future orientation), interpersonal skills, knowledge about and attitudes towards sex and contraception, previous sexual, contraceptive and pregnancy experiences, peer norms, relationship status and a situational variable – substance abuse prior to coitus. The model was tested using a sample of 283 male and female college students. Twenty-six-and-a-half per cent of the variance in the dependent measure was accounted for mainly by perceived barriers, contraceptive use at first coitus, past pregnancies and relationship status. The explained variance rose to 44.4 per cent for a subsample ($n = 95$) reporting current involvement with one partner where substance abuse prior to coitus entered the regression equation. Caution might again be appropriate in interpreting Lowe and Radius' findings since the authors do not report how their dichotomous dependent variable, 'effective' vs 'ineffective' contraceptive method used at last intercourse, was defined.

## Developmental models

The second group of theories of CU is developmental models. These theories focus on young people's developing psychosexual maturity, particularly that of young women, and view CU as a process which may be characterized by a number of stages. Progress through stages of one's contraceptive 'career' is motivated by increased sexual activity and a developing acceptance of one's sexuality. Lindemann's (1974, 1977) account posits three stages. In the first 'natural' stage, sexual intercourse is relatively rare and unplanned and the woman herself is unlikely to use contraception since she does not, as yet, see herself as sexual. The second 'peer-prescription' stage is characterized by seeking contraceptive information from close friends. Sexual intercourse is more frequent at this stage, although it is likely that less effective or coitus-dependent contraceptive methods are used, since sexual self-acceptance is only moderate at best. In the final 'expert' stage, the woman has incorporated sexuality into her self-concept and will seek professional advice and plan her contraceptive activity.

Rains' (1971) model specifies 'moral ambivalence' about sexual activity as the central motivating force in the transition from virginity to sexual activity and CU. Only when a woman accepts sexual activity as 'right for her' will she take responsibility for CU and progress beyond non-use or inconsistent use. Four stages characterize this process. The first stage is falling in love, which provides a rationale for sexual intimacy. The second stage involves an exclusive, and by implication, a stable or longer-term relationship with one man. In the third stage the woman comes to see sexual intercourse as acceptable for herself. By the fourth and final stage the woman has accepted her sexuality and sees herself as likely to have sexual intercourse in the future. Rains argues that it is this fourth stage that is most likely to produce consistent CU.

These developmental theories have received little empirical attention. Lindemann's account does not appear to have been tested while DeLamater and MacCorquodale's (1978) study is the only one that has examined Rains' (1971) model. Variables specified by Rains explained 16 per cent of the variance in female CU and 11 per cent of male use. Greater sexual activity and discussion of contraception were significant predictors for both groups, although the exclusivity of the sexual relationship was also an important predictor of female CU.

Another account of CU which incorporates elements of both decision making and developmental perspectives is that of DeLamater (1983). Like Lindemann, DeLamater sees increasing frequency of sexual intercourse in terms of both relative frequency with current partner and number of lifetime coital experiences as the prime mover in the development of CU. Frequency of intercourse is believed to be a function of both the intimacy of the relationship and the person's sexual standards. With increasing sexual activity the possibility of pregnancy is considered and cognitive assessment of the costs/benefits of pregnancy takes place. On the basis of this assessment a decision about CU is made. Experiences with contraception, positive or negative, then feed back to influence the central variable, frequency of intercourse. While several studies support associations proposed by DeLamater, the formulation in its entirety has not been empirically tested. It is worth noting, however, that the path analytic study of Herold and McNamee (1982) did not support the central mediating role of intercourse frequency which characterizes each of the developmental models outlined above.

**Summary**

Comparisons between the models outlined above are difficult because of the wide variation in samples used and differences in the operationalization of the dependent variable. It is worth noting, moreover, that developmental and decision models have different focuses and should be considered complementary rather than competing frameworks. Decision models focus upon individual

differences in CU while developmental models are more concerned with changes
in a single individual's CU over time. In this respect, decision models are
probably more amenable to quantitative research and have consequently
received greater attention in the literature. What is required, however, is greater
integration of variables specified by both frameworks in a single unified account.
It would seem apparent that more eclectic models have been the most successful
in predicting CU (e.g. Fisher's test of Byrne's model, 1984; Herold and
McNamee, 1982; Lowe and Radius, 1987). A balanced conception of both
intrapersonal (attitudes, beliefs, knowledge, personality) and interpersonal
(partner, parents, peers, situations) factors is therefore required in order to
develop a more comprehensive theory of CU. In the next section, research
findings with respect to five groups of variables – background factors;
knowledge, attitudes and beliefs; interpersonal factors, personality factors
and situational factors – are summarized.

# Factors associated with contraceptive use:
# a synthesis of findings

## Background factors

Because samples employed in research on CU are generally both small and
non-random, not a great deal of research has been conducted on background
variables such as age, gender, race, socio-economic status (SES) or education.
Most studies find that young women's CU increases with age (e.g. Herold,
1981b; Furstenburg, Shea, Allison et al., 1983; Zelnik and Kanter, 1977),
although this finding may be limited to non-student samples (Hill, Peplau and
Rubin, 1983; DeLamater and MacCorquodale, 1979). Whitely and Schofield
(1986) in a meta-analysis of 134 studies found a small but significant relationship between gender and whether or not contraception was used (mean $r = 0.08$
across twenty studies). The mean $r$ was higher in the case of five studies which
examined whether respondents *themselves* had used contraception (mean
$r = 0.28$). Not surprisingly, being female was associated with greater CU than
being male. Small but significant effects of race were also obtained by Whitely
and Schofield. Across seventeen North American studies a mean $r$ of 0.08 with
CU was observed, with whites slightly more likely to use contraception than
blacks. The effects of race, moreover, did not appear to vary as a function of
gender.

Hornick, Doran and Crawford (1979) found a significant positive effect of
SES upon female but not male CU. Other studies found no effect of SES
although this may be due to the consideration that the distribution of SES scores
were probably quite attenuated among the samples employed (e.g. Foreit and
Foreit, 1978; Herold, 1981b; Jones and Phillibur, 1983). There is little evidence
to suggest that Catholics, Protestants and Jews differ significantly in their CU
(Garris, Steckler and McIntyre, 1976; Hill, Peplau and Rubin, 1983; Kanter and
Zelnik, 1973) or that religiosity is substantially correlated with CU (Herold,
1981b; DeLamater and MacCorquodale, 1979; Rosen and Ager, 1981). School
performance was significantly associated with CU among high-school women in
Furstenburg, Shea, Allison et al.'s (1983) study although Foreit and Foreit (1978)
did not find a significant relationship among bright college students. Higher

educational aspirations are also positively and significantly associated with CU (Herold and Samson, 1980; Shah, Zelnik and Kanter, 1975; Jones and Phillibur, 1983).

The effects of background variables on CU are generally small. Lowe and Radius (1987) found that the six variables mentioned above accounted for just 2 per cent of the variance in their CU measure. What little effect background variables have may be largely indirect. There is a great deal of evidence which suggests that age, gender, race, SES, and education influence knowledge and attitudes about sex and contraception and that these variables in turn influence CU (DeLamater and MacCorquodale, 1979; DelCampo, Sporakawski and DelCampo, 1976; Lieberman, 1981; Finkel and Finkel, 1975; Reichelt and Werely, 1975; Sheeran, Abraham, Abrams et al., 1990; Zelnik and Kanter, 1977). Background variables might also be important in moderating the effects of sexual self-acceptance, attitudes or other psychological variables on CU. Kastner (1984), for example, found a larger correlation between parental support and CU among 15/16-year olds than 17/18-year olds ($rs = 0.56$ and $0.20$). Unfortunately, few if any other studies appears to have used this moderator variable perspective.

### Knowledge, attitudes and beliefs

Adequate information about sex, pregnancy and contraception must be a pre-requisite of contraceptive decision making. Even research published during the 1980s, however, shows that a number of startling errors of fact seems to characterize young people's knowledge in this areas. Ten per cent of Cvetkovich and Grote's (1981) subjects did not believe that they could become pregnant the first time they had sexual intercourse while 52 per cent of men and 37 per cent of women could not identify the period of greatest pregnancy risk during the menstrual cycle (see also DeAmicis, Klorman, Hess and McAnarney, 1981). Two-fifths of respondents in Lowe and Radius' (1987) study did not know how long sperm remains viable. More than 12 per cent did not think it was necessary to hold a condom when withdrawing while 20.6 per cent did not know it was essential to use spermicide with the diaphragm. These findings are all the more disturbing since such knowledge is demonstrably related to CU. Whitely and Schofield (1986) found a mean correlation of 0.17 between CU and objective knowledge tests among both men and women across twenty-five studies.

Accumulated research evidence strongly supports the view that more positive contraceptive attitudes are associated with increased CU (Fisher, 1984; Gerrard, McCann and Fortini, 1983; Hendricks and Fullilive, 1983; Herold and Goodwin, 1981; Herold and McNamee, 1982). An important line of research with implications for educational intervention has been the investigation of those beliefs which maintain negative contraceptive attitudes. Beliefs about contra-ception reducing the spontaneity of sex is cited as a reason for contraceptive non-use by 16.9 per cent of women and 32 per cent of men while 12 per cent of women and 25 per cent of men cite the belief that contraception is 'too much trouble to use' (Whitely and Schofield, 1986). Concerns about negative side effects, particularly in relation to oral contraceptives, are also noted in several studies (e.g. Jaccard and Davidson, 1972; Werner and Middlestadt, 1979; Boyce and Benoit, 1975; Herold and Goodwin, 1981).

Different standards for male and female sexual activity still persist (Spears, Abrams, Sheeran et al., 1991) and may be the basis of some negative beliefs about contraception. In the study by Freeman, Rickets, Mudd and Higgins (1981) two-thirds of the female respondents said that a girl would feel 'used' if her partner knew that she used contraception. Similarly, 17 per cent of Lowe and Radius' (1987) sample believed that females with accessible contraception would be deemed promiscuous while 31 per cent believed that accessible contraception would 'make it too easy' to have intercourse.

## Intrapersonal factors

Interactions with partner, parent and peers are important sources of information about contraception and important influences on CU. DeLamater and MacCorquodale (1979) found that men rated their partners as the most important source of contraceptive information while professionals such as doctors and clergy were rated highest by women. Parents were the least important source for both men and women. Vincent, Falkenberry and Murray (1981) found that mass media and advice from friends were equally cited as the most important information source among their mixed-sex sample. A previous study by Vincent and Stelling (1973), however, found that 64 per cent of all respondents received their knowledge from reading on their own, with physicians being ranked second by women and advice from friends the next most important source for both groups.

*Partner:* According to developmental models, characteristics of the relationship between sexual partners should be an important predictor of CU. The weight of research evidence supports the view that characteristics such as duration (Cole, Beighton and Jones, 1975; Cvetkovich and Grote, 1981; Foreit and Foreit, 1981), intimacy (Furstenburg, Shea, Allison et al., 1983; Hornick, Doran and Crawford, 1979) type of relationship operationalized in terms such as casual vs steady vs engaged (Fujita, Wagner and Pion, 1971; Furstenburg, 1971; MacCance and Hall, 1972) and especially exclusivity (DeLamater and MacCorquodale, 1978; Herold and McNamee, 1982; Reichelt, 1979; Thompson and Spanier, 1978) are each positively and significantly associated with CU. Another relationship variable which may perhaps mediate the influence of the characteristics outlined above is frequency of intercourse (DeLamater, 1983). Virtually all studies find that intercourse frequency is positively related to CU (Cvetkovich and Grote, 1981; Foreit and Foreit, 1978, 1981; Geis and Gerrard, 1984; Herold, 1981b; Thompson and Spanier, 1978).

Overt discussion of birth control between sexual partners is very reliably associated with both consistency and effectiveness of CU (Herold and McNamee, 1982; Herold and Samson, 1980; Jorgensen, King and Torrey, 1980; Jones and Phillibur, 1983). Discussion of contraception is also positively related to intercourse frequency (Vincent and Stelling, 1973). A number of studies suggest that partner influence to use contraception might be more important than discussion *per se* (Cohen and Rose, 1984; Cvetkovich and Grote, 1981; Kastner, 1984). Herold and McNamee's (1982) path analytic study obtained a significant direct path between partner influence and CU. Whitely and Schofield (1986) found large mean correlations between partner influence and CU for both men and women. The mean $r$s were 0.35 for women and 0.51 for men across seven and three studies respectively.

*Parents:* The quality of the person's relationship with their parents does not appear to be a significant factor in CU (Cahn, 1978; DeLamater and MacCorquodale, 1979; Jones and Phillibur, 1983; Oskamp and Mindick, 1983). Parents' greater sexual permissiveness, however, has been shown to be positively related to CU in a number of studies (Furstenburg, 1971; Cahn, 1978; Hornick, Doran and Crawford, 1979). Explicit communication about contraception between mothers and daughters may also be a factor in encouraging women's CU (Furstenburg, 1971; Herold and Samson, 1980) although a number of studies do not support this relationship (Reiss, Banwart and Foreman, 1975; Thompson and Spanier, 1978). Fathers appear to have little or no influence upon their childrens' contraceptive behaviour (Milan and Kilmann, 1987).

*Peers:* Peer permissiveness regarding sexual activity has been negatively correlated with contraceptive embarrassment (Herold, 1981b) and positively correlated with contraceptive use (Herold and McNamee, 1982). Perceived peer attitudes towards contraception do not appear to influence women's CU (Jorgensen, 1980; Jorgensen and Sonstegard, 1984). However, peers' sexual and contraceptive behaviour may be a factor in both use vs non-use (DeLamater and MacCorquodale, 1979; Jorgensen, 1980; Herold and Samson, 1980) and use of a more reliable method (Venham, 1972, cited in Milan and Kilmann, 1987). Peer influence to use contraception may also be an important predictor of women's contraceptive behaviour. Herold and Samson (1980) found that virgin teenage girls who had discussed pill use more frequently with their friends were more likely to obtain oral contraception before rather than after first intercourse. There is little evidence on the relationship between peer discussion or influence and male CU although it appears that such communications are less frequent among men and are consequently less relevant to their contraceptive behaviours.

## Personality influences

Several researchers have demonstrated relationships between personality variables and CU. Low levels of socialization – that is, incomplete learning and/or acceptance of societal norms – are related to both use of an unreliable contraceptive method and to inconsistent CU (Gough, 1973a and b; Oskamp and Mindick, 1983). Similarly CU is negatively related to measures of conservatism (Lundy, 1972; Geis and Gerrard, 1984) and to sex-role traditionality (Fox, 1977; DeLamater and MacCorquodale, 1979; McCormick, Izzo and Folcik, 1985).

Locus of control and self-esteem have been extensively investigated although findings with respect to these variables are somewhat contradictory. Morrison (1985) argues that while internal locus of control is positively related to use vs non-use, there is no relationship with choice of birth control. Since locus of control is a general construct it may be the case that more sexually specific measures of efficacy would correlate more highly with CU (Rotter, 1975). Empirical research does appear to support this view (Brown, 1977; Grunebaum and Abernathy, 1974). Most studies find little or no relationship between self-esteem and CU (Lundy, 1972; Garris et al., 1976; DeLamater and MacCorquodale, 1979). However, there appears to be a significant effect for self-esteem on contraceptive behaviours that involve FP clinic attendance (Reiss, Banwart and Foreman, 1975; Herold, Goodwin and Lero, 1979). It is worth noting that Whitely and Schofield (1986) found no evidence to suggest that self-esteem or locus of control are predictive of male contraceptive behaviour.

A number of cognitive variables have also received attention. While there is little evidence to suggest that IQ scores are related to CU (Brown, 1977; Oskamp, Mindick, Berger and Motta, 1978) significant associations have been observed for problem-solving ability (Steinlauf, 1979) and measures of planfulness including future orientation and impulse control (Berlanger and Bradley, 1971; Harvey, 1976; Jones and Phillibur, 1983). Neither moral development (e.g. Jurs, 1984) nor risk-taking (e.g. Rader, Bekker, Brown and Richardt, 1978), however, have demonstrated significant relationships.

A final group of personality variables which have proven successful in predicting CU relate to dispositions to respond positively or negatively to sexual cues. These include erotophilia–erotophobia, mentioned earlier, sex guilt and sex anxiety. Erotophilia–erotophobia is positively related to attitudes and norms about birth control as well as behaviours such as clinic attendance and consistency of CU (Fisher, Byrne, Edmunds et al., 1979; Fisher, 1984). Studies using measures of sex guilt have also found significant associations with both use vs non-use and consistency of use (Lehfeldt, 1971; Gerrard, 1982; Upchurch, 1978; Herold and McNamee, 1982). Gerrard (1977) found that these relationships with sex guilt held for users of each of the major contraceptive methods.

There is evidence to suggest that both trait (Joesting and Joesting, 1974) and state anxiety (Brooks and Butcalis, 1976) but not neuroticism (Oskamp, Mindick, Berger and Motta, 1978) are related to CU. Leary and Dobbins (1983) altered a standard social anxiety scale so that it measured *heterosocial* anxiety or anxiety experienced in social interactions with the opposite sex. They found that heterosocial anxiety was positively associated with women's relying on their male partners to use condoms and was negatively associated with use of oral contraception or the diaphragm. More specific measures of sex anxiety such as the scale developed by Janda and O'Grady (1980) have also been successful in predicting contraceptive practice (Burger and Inderbitzen, 1985; Herold and McNamee, 1982).

## Situational factors

While the potential importance of situational factors is acknowledged by most researchers few studies have incorporated situational variables in their analyses. One exception is Herold and McNamee's (1982) study which found a correlation of 0.34 between substance abuse prior to coitus and CU among respondents reporting current involvement with one partner. Another situational variable, living at home vs away from home, is also related to CU. Greater use of contraception is associated with living away from home for both women (Kanter and Zelnik, 1973) and men (Hill, Peplau and Rubin, 1983) although this may be because of greater intercourse frequency or because there is less fear of parental discovery or sanction.

Studies reporting reasons for non-use of contraception provide most evidence for the importance of situational factors although it should be noted that these are

**Table 8.2** Percentage of respondents citing situational factors as reasons for non-use of contraception

| Reason | % | No. of studies |
|---|---|---|
| Unplanned intercourse | 38.0 | 17 |
| Intercourse during safe period | 30.8 | 11 |
| Did not think about pregnancy | 26.0 | 1 |
| Perceived non-availability | 17.4 | 5 |
| Didn't know where to get | 12.9 | 12 |
| Impression management | 10.2 | 4 |
| High financial cost | 7.5 | 3 |
| 'Don't care' if pregnancy results | 7.5 | 3 |

Based on a reanalysis of data presented by Whitely and Schofield (1986)

retrospective accounts and may be subject to memory or self-serving biases. Table 8.2 presents the percentages of respondents citing situational factors for non-use of contraception.

Spontaneous sexual intercourse appears to be the major factor in contraceptive non-use and is cited by almost two-fifths of respondents. One-tenth said they did not want to use contraception because they did not want to give the impression that intercourse had been planned. The potential significance of sexual arousal (see Byrne, 1983) may perhaps be indicated by the percentage of respondents endorsing thoughtlessness or 'don't care' as reasons for non-use. Unfortunately, little or no experimental research has been conducted to clarify the influence of this variable.

Incomplete knowledge about the 'safe' period or lack of attention to stages of the menstrual cycle may be implicated in the reason given by almost one-third of respondents – that they thought that they had had intercourse during the safe period. Situational factors related to obtaining contraception such as perceived non-availability, high cost and information on the location of clinics are also important. Phipps-Yonas (1980) points out that factors such as interactions with FP clinic staff and distance from the clinic may also contribute to contraceptive risk-taking. Rokeach's (1972) attitude model represents one potentially useful perspective within which situational factors can be accommodated. His model specifically holds that behaviour is a *joint* function of both attitudes towards the behaviour and attitudes towards the situation in which the behaviour occurs.

## Summary

Since studies generally do not operationalize variables from each of the five categories outlined above it is not appropriate to compare variables across categories. In general, however, background variables such as age, gender, SES, etc. have small but significant effects on CU. The influence of these variables may be more important in terms of their indirect influence on knowledge and attitudes. Knowledge and attitudes about sex and contraception have highly reliable effects on contraceptive behaviour. Partners are the most important interpersonal factor in CU with frequency of intercourse and partner influence to use contraception the most significant individual variables. Personality variables specifically concerned with emotional responses to sexuality such as erotophilia–erotophobia, sex guilt and sex anxiety are also reliably associated with

CU. Situational factors have largely been neglected by quantitative researchers although spontaneity of intercourse and perceived non-availability appear to have important influences on non-use.

## Conclusion

Although psychological factors have been extensively studied in relation to premarital contraceptive use, the wide variety of operationalizations of CU and the absence of a coherent conceptual framework within which to integrate findings make it difficult to assess our cumulative knowledge in this area. While most of the extant theoretical frameworks find some empirical support, in general, the explained variance in the dependent measure is only between 20 and 30 per cent. A more unified theoretical framework is required that incorporates elements of both decision making and developmental accounts. It is important also that this framework draws from each of the five variable categories – background, knowledge and attitudes, interpersonal, personality and situational – outlined above.

At the level of sampling, more frequent use of random samples and greater attention to the determinants of male contraceptive behaviour are desirable. This latter consideration is particularly important in the context of AIDS since contraception may be becoming either more male-orientated or more of a joint decision-making process. Further research is required on sexually active young people in order to determine whether consideration of infection by HIV is of equal or greater importance than pregnancy avoidance in contraceptive decisions being made today.

## Applications

### 1. Developmental and decision-making aspects
The psychological models of contraceptive use suggest that it is not just a decision-making process but also a developmental one. An individual may change their contraceptive behaviour or choice of contraception as they change over time and as their circumstances change.

### 2. Psychological and situational factors
Practitioners should be aware that psychological factors do not predict contraceptive use very well on their own. In other words, it is not true to say that some young people are of a contraceptive-using type and others are not. Situational factors are particularly important in non-use of contraception, particularly spontaneous or unplanned sex and non-availability of contraceptives.

### 3. Interpersonal factors
Most research on contraceptive use, and most contraceptive advice, focuses on individuals. It is important to recognize that contraceptive use is an interpersonal activity. Relationship dynamics are important determinants of contraceptive use, not just in terms of intercourse frequency and the stability of the relationship, but also in terms of the ability of couples to talk about sex and to assert and act on their own needs and wishes. Contraceptive advice may be more effective if directed at couples. Similarly, adolescents may be more able to use contraception if they have opportunities to develop and practise negotiation skills in a 'safe' setting.

## Further reading

Walker, A. and McNeill, E. (eds) (1991). Family Planning and Reproductive Decisions: Theme Issues of the *Journal of Reproductive and Infant Psychology*, **9**, 4, 215–69.
Homans, H. (ed.) (1985). *The Sexual Politics of Reproduction*. Aldershot: Gower.

## References

Alan Guttmacher Institute (1981). *Teenage Pregnancy: The Problem Hasn't Gone Away*. New York: Alan Guttmacher Institute.
Beck, J. G. and Davies, D. K. (1982). Teen contraception: a review of perspectives on compliance. *Archives of Sexual Behaviour*, **16**, 337–68.
Berlanger, K. and Bradley, E. J. (1971). Two groups of university student women: sexual activity and the use of contraception. *Journal of the American College Health Association*, **19**, 307–12.

Boyce, J. and Benoit, C. (1975). Adolescent pregnancy. *New York State Journal of Medicine*, **75**, 872–4.

Brooks, G. G. and Butcalis, M. R. (1976). Psychometric testing as a basis for counselling patients choosing a method of contraception. *American Journal of Obstetrics and Gynecology*, **124**, 85–7.

Brown, L. S. (1977). Do users have more fun: a study of the relationship between contraceptive behaviour, sexual assertiveness, and patterns of causal attribution. Unpublished doctoral dissertation, Southern Illinois University at Carbondale.

Burger, J. M. and Inderbitzen, H. M. (1985). Predicting contraceptive behaviour among college students: the role of communication, knowledge, sexual anxiety and self-esteem. *Archives of Sexual Behaviour*, **14**, 343–50.

Byrne, D. (1983). Sex without contraception. In *Adolescents, Sex, and Contraception* (D. Byrne and W. A. Fisher, eds). Hillsdale, NJ: Erlbaum.

Byrne, D., Jazwinski, C., DeNinno, J. A. and Fisher, W. A. (1977). Negative sexual attitudes and contraception. In *Exploring Human Sexuality* (D. Byrne and L. A. Byrne, eds). New York: Crowell.

Cahn, J. (1978). The influence of others on teenagers' use of birth control (Doctoral Dissertation, City University of New York, 1978). *Dissertation Abstracts International*, **39**, 1537B.

Chilman, C. S. (1983). *Adolescent Sexuality in a Changing American Society*. 2nd edn, New York: Wiley.

Cohen, D. D. and Rose, R. D. (1984). Male adolescent birth control behaviour: the importance of developmental factors and sex differences. *Journal of Youth and Adolescence*, **13**, 239–52.

Cohen, J. B., Severy, L. J. and Ahtola, O. T. (1978). An extended expectancy–value approach to contraceptive alternatives. *Journal of Population*, **1**, 22–41.

Cole, J. B., Beighton, F. C. L. and Jones, I. H. (1975). Contraceptive practice and unplanned pregnancy among single university students. *British Medical Journal*, **4**, 217–19.

Cvetkovich, G. and Grote, B. (1981). Psychosocial maturity and teenage contraceptive use: an investigation of decision-making and communication skills. *Population and Environment*, **4**, 211–26.

Davidson, A. R. and Jaccard, J. J. (1975). Population psychology: a new look at an old problem. *Journal of Personality and Social Psychology*, **31**, 1073–82.

DeAmicis, L. A., Klorman, R., Hess, D. W. and McAnarney, E. R. (1981). A comparison of unwed pregnant teenagers and nulligravid sexually active adolescents seeking contraception. *Adolescence*, **16**, 11–20.

DeLamater, J. (1983). An interpersonal and interactional model of contraceptive behaviour. In *Adolescents, Sex and Contraception* (D. Byrne and W. A. Fisher, eds) pp. 33–48. Hillsdale, NJ: Erlbaum.

DeLamater, J. and MacCorquodale, P. (1978). Premarital contraceptive use: a test of two models. *Journal of Marriage and the Family*, **40**, 235–47.

DeLamater, J. and MacCorquodale, P. (1979). *Premarital Sexuality: Attitudes, Relationships, Behaviour*. Madison, WI; University of Wisconsin Press.

DelCampo, R. L., Sporakowski, M. J. and DelCampo, D. S. (1976). Premarital sexual permissiveness and contraceptive knowledge: a biracial comparison of college students. *Journal of Sex Research*, **12**, 180–92.

Edwards, N. (1954). The theory of decision making. *Psychological Bulletin*, **51**, 380–417.

Ewald, B. M. and Roberts, C. S. (1981). Contraceptive behaviour in college age males related to the Fishbein model. *Advances in Nursing Science*, **7**, 63–9.

Finkel, M. L. and Finkel, D. J. (1975). Sexual and contraceptive knowledge, attitudes and behavior of male adolescents. *Family Planning Perspectives*, **7**, 256–60.

Finkel, M. L. and Finkel, D. J. (1983). Male adolescent sexual behaviour, the forgotton partner: a review. *Journal of School Health*, **53**, 544–7.

Fishbein, M. (1972). Toward an understanding of family planning behaviours. *Journal of Applied Social Psychology*, **2**, 214–27.

Fishbein, M. and Ajzen, I. (1975). *Belief, Attitude, Intention and Behaviour*. Reading, MA: Addison-Wesley.

Fishbein, M. and Jaccard, J. J. (1973). Theoretical and methodological considerations in the prediction of family planning intentions and behaviour. *Representative Research in Social Psychology*, **4**, 37–52.

Fisher, W. A. (1984). Predicting contraceptive behavior among university men: the role of emotions and behavioral intentions. *Journal of Applied Social Psychology*, **14**, 104–23.

Fisher, W. A., Byrne, D., Edmunds, M., Miller, C. T., Kelley, K. and White, L. A. (1979). Psychological and situation-specific correlates of contraceptive behavior among university women. *Journal of Sex Research*, **15**, 38–55.

Foreit, K. G. and Foreit, J. R. (1978). Correlates of contraceptive behavior among unmarried U.S. college students. *Studies in Family Planning*, **9**, 169–74.

Foreit, J. R. and Foreit, K. G. (1981). Risk-taking and contraceptive behavior among unmarried college students. *Population and Environment*, **4**, 174–88.

Fox, G. L. (1977). Sex-role attitudes as predictors of contraceptive use among unmarried university students. *Sex Roles*, **3**, 265–83.

Freeman, E. W., Rickets, K., Mudd, E. B. H. and Higgins, G. R. (1982). Never-pregnant adolescents and family planning programs: contraception, continuation, and pregnancy risk. *American Journal of Public Health*, **72**, 815–22.

Fujita, B. N., Wagner, N. N. and Pion, R. J. (1971). Contraceptive use among single college students. *American Journal of Obstetrics and Gynecology*, **109**, 787–93.

Furstenburg Jr, F. F. (1971). Preventing unwanted pregnancies among adolescents. *Journal of Health and Social Behavior*, **12**, 340–47.

Furstenburg Jr, F. F., Shea, J., Allison, P., Herceg-Baron, R. and Webb, D. (1983). Contraceptive continuation among adolescents attending family planning clinics. *Family Planning Perspectives*, **15**, 211–17.

Garris, L., Steckler, A. and McIntyre, J. R. (1976). The relationship between oral contraceptives and adolescent sexual behavior. *Journal of Sex Research*, **12**, 135–46.

Geis, B. D. and Gerrard, M. (1984). Predicting male and female contraceptive behavior: a discriminant analysis of groups high, moderate, and low in contraceptive effectiveness. *Journal of Personality and Social Psychology*, **46**, 669–80.

Gerrard, M. (1977). Sex guilt in abortion patients. *Journal of Consulting and Clinical Psychology*, **45**, 708.

Gerrard, M. (1982). Sex, sex guilt, and contraceptive use. *Journal of Personality and Social Psychology*, **42**, 153–8.

Gerrard, M., McCann, L. and Fortini, M. E. (1983). Prevention of unwanted pregnancy. *American Journal of Community Psychology*, **11**, 153–67.

Gough, H. G. (1973a). A factor analysis of contraceptive preferences. *Journal of Psychology*, **84**, 199–210.

Gough, H. G. (1973b). Personality assessment in the study of population. In *Psychological Perspectives on Population* (J. R. Fawcett, ed.). New York: Basic Books.

Grunebaum, H. and Abernathy, V. (1974). Marital decision making as applied to family planning. *Journal of Sex and Marital Therapy*, **1**, 63–74.

Harvey, A. L. (1976). Risky and safe contraception: some personality factors. *Journal of Psychology*, **92**, 109–12.

Hendricks, L. E. and Fullilive, R. E. (1983). Locus of control and the use of contraception among unmarried black adolescent fathers and their controls: a preliminary report. *Journal of Youth and Adolescence*, **12**, 225–33.

Herold, E. S. (1981a). Measurement issues involved in examining contraceptive use among young single women. *Population and Environment*, **4**, 128–44.

Herold, E. S. (1981b). Contraceptive embarrassment and contraceptive behavior among young single women. *Journal of Youth and Adolescence*, **10**, 233–42.

Herold, E. S. and Goodwin, M. S. (1981). Premarital sex guilt and contraceptive attitudes and behavior. *Family Relations*, **30**, 247–53.

Herold, E. S. and McNamee, J. E. (1982). An explanatory model of contraceptive use among young women. *Journal of Sex Research*, **18**, 289–304.

Herold, E. S. and Samson, M. (1980). Differences between women who begin pill use before and after first intercourse: Ontario, Canada. *Family Planning Perspectives*, **12**, 304–5.

Herold, E. S., Goodwin, M. S. and Lero, D. S. (1979). Self-esteem locus of control and adolescent contraception. *Journal of Psychology*, **101**, 83–8.

Hill, C. T., Peplau, L. A. and Rubin, Z. (1983). Contraceptive use by college dating couples: a comparison of men's and women's reports. *Population and Environment*, **6**, 60–9.

Hornick, J. P., Doran, L. and Crawford, S. H. (1979). Premarital contraceptive usage among male and female adolescents. *Family Coordinator*, **28**, 181–90.

Jaccard, J. J. and Davidson, A. R. (1972). Towards an understanding of family planning behaviors: an initial investigation. *Journal of Applied Social Psychology*, **2**, 228–35.

Janda, L. H. and O'Grady, K. E. (1980). Development of a sex anxiety inventory. *Journal of Consulting and Clinical Psychology*, **48**, 169–75.

Joesting, J. and Joesting, R. (1974). Correlations among women's views of contraception, anxiety, creativity and equalitarianism measures. *Journal of Psychology*, **86**, 49–51.

Jones, E. F., Forrest, J. D., Goldman, N., Henshaw, S. K., Lincoln, R., Rosoff, J. P., Westoff, C. F. and Wulf, D. (1985). Teenage pregnancy in developed countries: determinants and policy implications. *Family Planning Perspectives*, **17**, 53–63.

Jones, J. B. and Phillibur, S. (1983). Sexually active but not pregnant: a comparison of teens who risk and teens who plan. *Journal of Youth and Adolescence*, **12**, 235–51.

Jorgensen, S. R. (1980). Contraceptive attitude–behaviour consistency in adolescence. *Population and Environment*, **3**, 174–94.

Jorgensen, S. R. and Sonstegard, J. S. (1984). Predicting adolescent sexual and contraceptive behaviour: an application and test of the Fishbein model. *Journal of Marriage and the Family*, **46**, 43–55.

Jorgensen, S. R., King, S. L. and Torrey, B. A. (1980). Dyadic and social network influences on adolescent exposure to pregnancy risk. *Journal of Marriage and the Family*, **42**, 141–55.

Jurs, J. (1984). Correlation of moral development with use of birth control and pregnancy among teenage girls. *Psychological Reports*, **55**, 1009–10.

Kanter, J. F. and Zelnik, M. (1973). Contraception and pregnancy: experience of young unmarried women in the United States. *Family Planning Perspectives*, **5**, 21–35.

Kastner, L. S. (1984). Ecological factors predicting adolescent contraceptive use: implications for intervention. *Journal of Adolescent Health Care*, **5**, 79–86.

Leary, M. R. and Dobbins, S. E. (1983). Social anxiety, sexual behavior, and contraceptive use. *Journal of Personality and Social Psychology*, **45**, 1347–54.

Lehfeldt, H. (1971). Psychology of contraceptive failure. *Medical Aspects of Human Sexuality*, **5**, 68–77.

Lieberman, J. J. (1981). Locus of control as related to birth control knowledge, attitudes and practice. *Adolescence*, **16**, 1–10.

Lindemann, C. (1974). *Birth Control and Unmarried Young Women*. New York: Springer.

Lindemann, C. (1977). Factors affecting the use of contraception in the nonmarital context. In *Progress in Sexology* (R. Gemme and C. C. Wheeler, eds) pp. 397–408. New York: Plenum.

Lowe, C. S. and Radius, S. M. (1987). Young adults' contraceptive practices: an investigation of influences. *Adolescence*, **22**, 291–304.

Luker, K. (1975). *Taking Chances: Abortion and the Decision not to Contracept*. Berkeley, CA: University of California Press.

Lundy, J. R. (1972). Some personality correlates of contraceptive use among unmarried female college students. *Journal of Psychology*, **80**, 9–14.

Mauldin, W. B. and Segal, S. J. (1988). Prevalence of contraceptive use: trends and issues. *Studies in Family Planning*, **19**, 335–53.

McCance, C. and Hall, D. J. (1972). Sexual behaviour and contraceptive practice of unmarried female undergraduates at Aberdeen University. *British Medical Journal*, **2**, 694–700.

McCormick, N., Izzo, A. and Folcik, J. (1985). Adolescents' values, sexuality, and contraception in a rural New York county. *Adolescence*, **20**, 385–95.

Milan, R. J. and Kilmann, P. R. (1987). Interpersonal factors in premarital contraception. *Journal of Sex Research*, **23**, 289–321.

Morrison, D. M. (1985). Adolescent contraceptive behaviour: a review. *Psychological Bulletin*, **98**, 538–68.

Oskamp, S. and Mindick, B. (1983). Personality and attitudinal barriers to contraception. In *Adolescents, Sex and Contraception* (D. Byrne and W. A. Fisher, eds) pp. 65–108. Hillsdale, NJ: Erlbaum.

Oskamp, S., Mindick, B., Berger, D. and Motta, E. (1978). A longitudinal study of success versus failure in contraceptive planning. *Journal of Population*, **1**, 69–83.

Phipps-Yonas, S. (1980). Teenage pregnancy and motherhood: a review of the literature. *American Journal of Orthopsychiatry*, **50**, 403–31.

Rains, P. (1971). *Becoming an Unwed Mother*. Chicago: Aldine.

Rader, G. E., Bekker, L. D., Brown, L. and Richardt, C. (1978). Psychological correlates of unwanted pregnancy. *Journal of Abnormal Psychology*, **87**, 373–6.

Reichelt, P. A. (1979). Coital and contraceptive behaviour of female adolescents. *Archives of Sexual Behaviour*, **8**, 159–72.

Reichelt, P. A. and Werley, H. H. (1975). Contraception, abortion and venereal disease: teenagers' knowledge and the effect of education. *Family Planning Perspectives*, **7**, 83–8.

Reiss, I. L., Banwart, A. and Foreman, H. (1975). Premarital contraceptive usage: a study and some theoretical explorations. *Journal of Marriage and the Family*, **37**, 619–30.

Rokeach, M. (1972). Behaviour as a function of attitude-toward-object and attitude-toward-situation. *Journal of Personality and Social Psychology*, **22**, 194–201.

Rosen, R. H. and Ager, J. W. (1981). Self-concept and contraception: pre-conception decision-making. *Population and Environment*, **4**, 11–23.

Rosenstock, I. M. (1974). The health belief model and preventive health behaviour. *Health Education Monographs*, **2**, 354–86.

Rotter, J. B. (1975). Some problems and misconceptions related to the construct of internal versus external control of reinforcement. *Journal of Consulting and Clinical Psychology*, **48**, 56–67.

Schinke, S. P., Gilchrist, L. D. and Small, R. W. (1979). Preventing unwanted pregnancy: a cognitive–behavioural approach. *American Journal of Orthopsychiatry*, **49**, 81–8.

Shah, F., Zelnik, M. and Kanter, J. F. (1975). Unprotected intercourse among unwed teenagers. *Family Planning Perspectives*, **7**, 39–44.

Sheeran, P., Abraham, S. C. S., Abrams, D., Spears, R. and Marks, D. (1990). The post AIDS structure of students' attitudes to condoms: age, sex and experience of use. *Psychological Reports*, **66**, 614.

Spears, R., Abrams, D., Sheeran, P., Abraham, S. C. S. and Marks, D. (1991). Social judgements of sex and blame in the context of AIDS: gender and linguistic frame. *British Journal of Social Psychology*, **30**, 37–49.

Steinlauf, B. (1979). Problem-solving skills, locus of control, and the contraceptive effectiveness of young women. *Child Development*, **50**, 268–71.

Thompson, L. and Spanier, G. B. (1978). Influence of parents, peers, and partners on the contraceptive use of college men and women. *Journal of Marriage and the Family*, **40**, 481–92.

Upchurch, M. L. (1978). Sex guilt and contraceptive use. *Journal of Sex Education and Therapy*, **4**, 27–31.

Vincent, M. L., Faulkenberry, J. R. and Murray, D. (1981). Contraceptive patterns of college students who experienced early coitus. *Journal of School Health*, **51**, 667–72.

Vincent, M. L. and Stelling, F. H. (1973). A survey of contraceptive practices and attitudes of unwed college students. *Journal of the American College Health Association*, **21**, 257–63.

Werner, P. D. and Middlestadt, S. E. (1979). Factors in the use of oral contraceptives by young women. *Journal of Applied Social Psychology*, **9**, 537–47.

Whitley, B. E. and Schofield, J. W. (1986). A meta-analysis of research on adolescent contraceptive use. *Population and Environment*, **8**, 173–203.

Zelnik, M. and Kanter, J. F. (1977). Sexual and contraceptive experience of young unmarried women in the United States, 1976 and 1971. *Family Planning Perspectives*, **9**, 55–71.

# 9

# Psychological aspects of elective abortion

## Anne Walker

Contraception is based on the control of fertility before conception has occurred, or before an embryo is viable. Abortion is used as a means of fertility control after an unwanted pregnancy has become established. Abortions which occur spontaneously (miscarriages) and 'therapeutic' abortions performed because prenatal screening has detected an abnormality or deformity in the baby will be discussed in the next book of this series. Like contraception, abortion is now safer and more reliable than at any other time in history. It is also increasingly an emotive subject. The 'pro-life'/'pro-choice' debate is familiar, insoluble and ever more bitter. Why do women end their pregnancies? Are some women more likely to have an abortion than others? What are the psychological consequences of a pregnancy termination? How do health care professionals cope with abortion procedures? These questions are addressed by Anne Walker in this chapter.

## Introduction

Abortions can be broadly divided into three types: spontaneous, therapeutic and elective. Spontaneous abortions, often called miscarriages, are estimated to occur in one-fifth of all known pregnancies (Slade, 1994), although many other embryos may be lost before the woman is aware that she is pregnant. Therapeutic abortion and elective abortion both refer to the intentional termination of a known pregnancy by medical or surgical intervention. I am using the term therapeutic abortion to refer to pregnancies which are ended because prenatal screening has identified an abnormality in the fetus. Elective abortions, which are the subject of this chapter, are conducted because of perceived risks to woman's physical or mental health or to that of her family (see Table 9.1).

---

**Table 9.1** A woman's pregnancy may be terminated if two medical practitioners agree that:

(a) The pregnancy has not exceeded its twenty-fourth week and that the continuance of the pregnancy would involve risk, greater than if the pregnancy were terminated, of injury to the physical or mental health of the pregnant woman or any existing children of her family; or
(b) That the termination is necessary to prevent grave permanent injury to the physical or mental health of the pregnant woman; or
(c) That the continuance of the pregnancy would involve risk to the life of the pregnant woman, greater than if the pregnancy were terminated; or
(d) That there is a substantial risk that if the child were born it would suffer from such physical or mental abnormalities as to be seriously handicapped.

*The Major Clause of the Abortion Act 1967 as Amended by the Human Fertilisation and Embryology Act, 1990.*

The psychological literature concerning abortion in Britain and the USA has developed since the liberalization of legislation in the late 1960s and early 1970s. Abortion therefore appears to be a modern phenomenon. This is far from the case. Abortion is one of the oldest and most widely practised methods of preventing the birth of unwanted children (Williams, 1987). In this century, abortion, like childbirth (Tew, 1990) has been placed firmly in the control of the medical profession and taken out of the control of lay practitioners and women themselves. Hence, the psychological literature is concerned with a particular form of abortion, controlled by legislation and the medical profession, and practised within a particular social setting. It should not be assumed that the same psychological processes are implicated in other cultures or at other times in history.

The history of abortion and the multitude of different methods and techniques for procuring miscarriage are described by Shorter (1983). Prior to the nineteenth century, herbal preparations were the most widely used means of procuring abortion. Humoral theories of medicine considered it harmful for a woman to miss her period, hence emmenagogues – drugs with the reputed ability to restore menstruation – were administered both by doctors and by folk medicine. These were probably abortifacients but were not medically sanctioned if pregnancy was suspected. References to herbal remedies for procuring miscarriage can also be found. The success of these methods is largely unknown. Their potency and toxicity would vary from season to season and with method of preparation hence it is unlikely that they were used routinely or in large numbers, and death of the pregnant woman was probably a frequent side-effect.

During the nineteenth century relatively safe and reliable instrumental means of ending a pregnancy were developed. These, together with enhanced aseptic procedures, increased the popularity of abortion. By 1939, the Birkett Committee on Abortion, following a joint Ministry of Health and Home Office investigation, estimated that between 110 000 and 150 000 illegal abortions were performed each year in Britain (Pipes, 1986), and it is estimated that among urban women between 1900 and 1940, one pregnancy in four ended this way (Shorter, 1983). These estimates are supported by many anecdotal reports from midwives on the high frequency of abortion in the 1930s (Simms, 1974). The number of cases of septic abortions and perforated uteri seen in hospitals also increased during this time – but this represents only a small proportion of all the illegal abortions conducted. By the 1930s, the death rate from illegal abortion was probably between 1 and 2 per cent (Shorter, 1983). Despite the gruesome reports of back-street abortion butchery (Humphries, 1988), abortion was safe in the vast majority of cases, and certainly safer than it had been at any previous time in history.

After the second world war, doctors were becoming increasingly willing to 'bend the rules' and conduct abortions legally on therapeutic grounds, so that by 1961, about 2300 abortions were being conducted annually within the NHS (Pipes, 1986). An extensive private practice also developed for psychiatrists who were willing (for a fee) to agree that a woman was too mentally unstable to bear a child. The subsequent abortion could then appear to be legal, if extremely costly for the woman concerned.

This latter point is an important one, especially when the psychological effects of abortion are being considered in early, post-legalization studies. The need for a woman to establish that her mental health was too unstable to risk bearing a child in order to obtain an abortion may influence ratings on psychological assessments completed in these early studies. One of the respondents in Mary Pipes' study (1986) of abortion describes her consultation like this:

> The psychiatrist tried to make me say that I really wanted another baby and that was why I had become pregnant. That was, of course rubbish. I had to be very dramatic – tears and all – to convince him that this wasn't the case, that I might do myself in if I had to go through with it – although that part was untrue – that it would be totally unfair on the boys and me to have it, etc. All very upsetting.

Abortion was legalized in Britain by the Abortion Act in 1967 (see Table 9.1), subject to the agreement of two medical practitioners, and the USA by the Supreme Court ruling in the case of Roe versus Wade (1973).

## Attitudes towards abortion

Abortion both in Europe and the USA remains a controversial practice, because of the varying psychological constructions of abortion. If abortion is constructed as the murder of a human being, and murder is believed to be morally wrong, then abortion too will be seen as morally wrong. This essentially is the rhetoric used by 'pro-life' campaigners (Vayreda and Antaki, 1991). If abortion is constructed as an act which prevents damage to the woman by the birth of an unwanted child, then abortion becomes morally acceptable, as argued by the 'pro-choice' campaigners (Vayreda and Antaki, 1991).

Many other constructions of abortion are clearly possible, and in many cases these correlate with a wider set of attitudes and beliefs. Kristin Luker (1984) studied over 200 pro-life and pro-choice activists in the USA (predominantly women in both groups) and found differing views on gender, sex and parenthood between the two groups. Pro-life campaigners were more likely to believe that men are more naturally suited to the public arena, while women are more naturally suited to domesticity and motherhood; that the primary purpose of sex is procreation; and that married people should accept parenthood whenever it occurs. Pro-choice activists, on the other hand, were more likely to believe that men and women should have equal rights and responsibilities; that sex is more for pleasure than procreation; and that parenthood should be optional and planned. Hence, the debate about abortion reflects deeper divisions between these groups in their philosophy of life.

The association with beliefs about women and motherhood in particular is also seen in Mary Boyle's study of the political debates surrounding both the Abortion Act of 1967 and later attempts to change the legislation. For example, opponents of abortion in these debates tended to see childbirth and motherhood as natural and unproblematic for women whilst supporters of legal abortion recognize the problems that motherhood can bring (Boyle, 1992, 1993).

Attitudes towards abortion also vary according to individual circumstances and experiences. Green, Snowdon and Statham (1993) surveyed 1528 British women during the first trimester of pregnancy, asking them whether they agreed or disagreed with abortion in seven different situations. Only 0.7 per cent felt that abortion should not be available under any circumstances. At the other extreme, only 22 per cent felt that abortion should be available in all circumstances.

Whilst having been pregnant before did not influence their attitudes, women who had previously had an abortion were more pro-abortion than the others, whilst women who had previously had a miscarriage were less in favour of abortion. Age and level of education of these women were also significant factors – older women and women with more years of education were in favour of abortion in more circumstances than younger or less well-educated women.

## Characteristics of abortion seekers

### Social and demographic characteristics

In 1988, 1.6 million abortions were performed in the USA (Russo, Horn and Schwartz, 1992). The comparable figure for England and Wales is 183 798 (Boyle, 1992). These numbers have remained fairly stable since legalization. Psychologists have become concerned with the characteristics of women seeking abortion in an attempt to identify those women who are likely to become pregnant, and therefore intervene to reduce the number of unwanted pregnancies. As Boyle (1993) points out, this endeavour has increased the emphasis on abortion as an individual issue (particular types of women have abortions) rather than a social issue (particular circumstances make an abortion more likely).

In both America and Britain, the majority of women seeking abortion are young (under 20), and women from lower social classes and minority ethnic groups are overrepresented in comparison to the general population (Russo, Horn and Schwartz, 1992; Handy, 1982). Some caution should be adopted when interpreting these figures, however.

Smith (1993) in a study of teenage pregnancy in Tayside between 1980 and 1990, showed that the rate of pregnancy was 4–8 times higher in the more deprived areas of the region (identified by postal code), and that about a quarter of these pregnancies resulted in abortion. In the wealthier areas, two-thirds of teenage pregnancies resulted in abortions. So, more advantaged young women are less likely to become pregnant, and more likely to abort the baby if they do become pregnant, a finding also supported by American statistics (Russo, Horn and Schwartz, 1992). The higher proportion of less advantaged women amongst the abortion statistics does not imply that lower class women are more likely to have abortions, but simply that more of them become pregnant in the first place. The decision to abort may be quite rational given their economic circumstances and employment prospects (Phoenix, 1991).

The larger proportion of young women having abortions has resulted in an emphasis on the 'problems' of teenage pregnancy. Older women also terminate their pregnancies on occasion. Russo, Horn and Schwartz (1992) surveyed 9480 women obtaining abortions at 103 clinics, hospitals and doctors' offices in the USA in 1987. Approximately one-third of this sample were over 25 years, and almost half of the total sample were already mothers. It is clear from their study that abortion is not simply used by women to avoid parental responsibility, but also to space children and limit the ultimate size of their families.

### Psychological characteristics

Are women who seek abortions psychologically different from those who do not? Abortion seekers have been shown to be more neurotic (Beard, Belsey, Lai et al., 1974), more depressed or anxious (Ford, Castelnuovo-Tedesco and Long,

1972), to display more deviant behaviours (Costa, Jessor and Donovan, 1987), and to have higher hypomania scores on the Minnesota Multiphasic Personality Inventory (Baetson, Rankin, Fuller et al., 1985) than pregnant women who are not seeking termination. Posavac and Miller (1990) suggest that the two groups may differ on a dimension of 'planfulness' – aborters may be less in control of their own lives. The validity of these studies is however impaired by the methodological difficulties which surround this area. Who should be included in the comparison group? A group of women carrying their babies to term may differ from an abortion seeking group on many confounding dimensions – the degree of intendedness of the pregnancy for instance, use of contraception and the social circumstances surrounding their pregnancy. In both cases, the psychological state of the woman at the time at which an abortion is being considered may not be the same as her pre-pregnancy state, hence it is difficult to know how these results could be meaningful as predictors of women likely to choose abortion.

Smetana and Adler (1979) tested Fishbein's model of behavioural intention (Fishbein and Ajzen, 1975) with women in the very early stages of a possible pregnancy. Women were asked what they would do if they were pregnant before they received the results of a pregnancy test, and as the model predicts, those who stated an intention to terminate the pregnancy were more likely to do so. The intention itself was predicted by the woman's beliefs about the expectations of significant others (e.g. partner, family, clergy) and her beliefs about the consequences of having a child. It would seem from this study that the decision to have an abortion is made relatively quickly, at a very early stage of the pregnancy and is based on the woman's perception of her circumstances and the views of the people around her before she even knows that she is pregnant.

A more specific theoretical model has been developed by Miller (1992) based on a review of the literature and a longitudinal study of 967 women in the San Francisco Bay area. This model includes five factors which are hypothesized to predict the decision to abort or not. It predicts that a woman is more likely to choose an abortion if she did not intend to become pregnant on the occasion of conception, if she is unable or unwilling to alter her life to accommodate a child, if she is not opposed to abortion on moral or religious grounds, and if abortion is readily available. In addition, the decision will be influenced by the time constraints and legal deadlines surrounding abortion and the views of the woman's partner, husband or family. Hence, the model places more emphasis on the social and situational circumstances of the woman than her personality characteristics. In the longitudinal study described by Miller, this model accounted for between 39 and 64 per cent of the variance in the decision to abort or not (depending on which cohort was sampled). Clearly, further testing is needed with independent samples, but this evidence suggests that women have abortions in particular circumstances, not that there is a particular type of woman who consistently chooses an abortion.

# Making the decision to have an abortion

## Individual decision making

There may be any number of psychological, practical and social factors which will predict on a large scale whether a woman will terminate her pregnancy or not. This information is of practical use to health educators and those concerned with preventing unwanted pregnancies from occurring. For the counsellor or clinician concerned with women seeking abortions, it is the process of decision making which is of more concern. Having discovered that she is pregnant, how does a woman decide whether to terminate or keep the pregnancy? How difficult is that decision and, if it is difficult, who might be able to help and how? From an academic point of view, studying how women decide whether or not to terminate a pregnancy provides useful real-life insight into decision making and developmental psychology (e.g. Gilligan, 1982).

The studies in this area can be divided into two categories – those which are concerned with the reasons given for choosing or not choosing an abortion (usually after the event), and those concerned with the process of making the decision. Both categories acknowledge that the decision itself is multifaceted, complex, and may be time consuming (Miller, 1992).

### Reasons for choosing an abortion

These studies are essentially descriptive and atheoretical. As with any study based on retrospective account giving, the participants are constructing a story of their feelings and experience which is acceptable both to themselves and to the researcher. Social cognition processes of impression management and causal attribution will therefore influence these findings (see Fiske and Taylor, 1991, for social cognition theory), as will the representations of abortion in a particular culture. Russo, Horn and Schwartz (1992) provide an analysis of the reasons given by 1900 abortion clients in a study by Torres and Forrest (1988). The reasons could be categorized into two broad types which they called personal/internal and situational/external. Internal reasons were to do with the woman's own personal qualities at the time, e.g. being 'too young' or immature for the responsibility of a baby. External reasons were to do with the situation in which the woman found herself, e.g. economic status, relationships with others, the health of the fetus/baby or commitments to education or work. Both external and internal reasons were important for all groups of women studied, but 75 per cent of the younger women (under 18) felt that their own psychological immaturity was a major reason for their decision.

### Process of decision making

The decision to have an abortion may be made very quickly, even before a woman is sure that she is pregnant (Allen, 1981; Cohan, Dunkel-Schetter and Lydon, 1993). An understanding of the process of decision making is however important for those who are counselling the women who experience more difficulty. Surprisingly, whilst there has been a great deal of research concerned with the psychological consequences of an abortion, very few studies have addressed the decision-making process, even though the degree of difficulty experienced with the decision has been shown to predict psychological outcome (Adler, David, Major et al., 1990).

Bracken, Klerman, Bracken et al., (1978a and b) used the Janis-Mann model of decision making as a theoretical base in a study of 498 never married women making their first visit to a prenatal clinic. Half of this group had decided to terminate the pregnancy, and the other half were matched to them on socio-demographic variables. The Janis-Mann model identifies five stages in the decision-making process:

1. Acknowledgement of the problem,
2. Formulation of alternative outcomes,
3. Consideration of the costs and benefits of various options,
4. Commitment to one choice over another, and
5. Adherence to the decision in the face of new information.

It was found that conflict could occur at any of these stages for the women, and that a variety of conflict resolution strategies were used. For example, all of the women were sad when they first suspected pregnancy, and in both groups denial of pregnancy was adopted as a coping strategy for about three weeks. Social support was also used as a coping strategy for women who experienced conflict at Stage 3 of the process. Here it was found that women who subsequently aborted discussed their pregnancy less frequently with significant others than those delivering. This may have been a self-protection strategy for them since women who later reported not having discussed their abortion with significant others were more satisfied with their decision to abort than those who had. The conclusions of this study were that although the decision making if an unplanned pregnancy occurs is not inconsequential, it is not necessarily conflictual for all women, and that subtle and crucial differences are seen between women, regardless of demographic characteristics. Those who do experience conflict adopt a variety of coping strategies at different stages, any of which may be appropriate (e.g. denial of the pregnancy may help to 'buy' thinking time). Problems did emerge for women, though, if external time constraints and/or coercion from significant others did not allow them to complete their own decision-making process. The authors suggest that counsellors need to identify the stage of the process which the woman has reached and design any intervention appropriately.

Carol Gilligan (1982) has placed abortion decision making within a developmental context. Her in-depth study of twenty-four pregnant women who were undecided about abortion at the time of the first interview, considered the process within the theoretical context of individual moral development. All of the women in this study were experiencing conflict over whether to terminate the pregnancy or not, and their resolution of the real-life dilemma was compared to the resolution of an artificial moral dilemma. The resolution of the real-life dilemma both depended on and reflected the stage of moral development which the woman had reached. At the earlier stages of development women give priority to self-preservation. With increasing maturity, responsibility for others (at the expense of personal safety) becomes more important. At the most mature stage, women are able to balance responsibility for others with a responsibility for themselves. The conflict experienced by an individual woman, and the way she resolves it depends upon her perception of what is right at that particular developmental stage. Although this study is based on a very small sample of women, with the purpose of elucidating women's moral development, it does make the important point that decision making about abortion is not independent of other psychological and developmental processes, which need to be taken account of in the counselling situation.

**Professional decision making**

In British law, the decision that an abortion should be conducted rests not with the pregnant woman, but with the doctors she consults, since two doctors must agree that the continued pregnancy would be more risky to her than a termination. A woman can only decide to ask for an abortion. The likelihood of that request being denied varies dramatically according to the woman's location. For instance, in 1988, only 1 per cent of the pregnancy terminations carried out on women living within the district of south Birmingham were conducted within the NHS, compared to 99 per cent of the terminations in north Devon (Coote, Harman and Hewitt, 1990). How do clinicians make this decision? Comments from women who had had abortions in Mary Pipes' study suggest that personal feelings may influence the judgement of some doctors:

> The consultant gynaecologist at the hospital was offensive, rude and obviously anti-abortion, although he did consent to the termination on the grounds that if he didn't, 'She'd only go off and pay £100 for it elsewhere'.

There is very little empirical research to support this experience however. Hamill and Ingram (1974) studied a group of women referred for psychiatric opinion on termination. They found that those granted a termination were older, more likely to be married and have children already, more likely to say that they had used contraception regularly, and to be rated as showing psychiatric symptoms, than those denied an abortion. Whether these findings reflect bias in clinical judgements or real differences in risk levels between the groups is difficult to assess, especially since the study was conducted twenty years ago. Clearly, further research is needed to investigate the decision making of clinicians in abortion consultations.

## The abortion procedure

Most medical and surgical procedures evoke anxiety which may be reduced by appropriate psychological interventions, e.g. cognitive coping strategies (Rafferty, 1993). Up to twelve weeks of gestation, vacuum aspiration is the technique most commonly used, although medical abortion techniques are becoming more common. Later abortions can be performed either using intra-amniotic methods (equivalent to inducing labour and delivering a dead fetus) or by dilatation and extraction (in which the cervix is dilated and the fetus removed). The risks, side effects and psychological aspects of these procedures might be expected to vary. As Handy (1982) points out, the choice of procedure is usually based on medical grounds without regard to the stressfulness of particular procedures for individual women. Osofsky and Osofsky (1972) found that approximately one-third of women awaiting suction termination were fearful of the procedure, suggesting that psychological intervention might be appropriate for this group.

The procedure of pregnancy termination may be stressful not only for the woman concerned, but also for the medical and nursing staff (Broome, 1984). As for pregnant women, some procedures may be more distressing for staff than others. Kaltreider, Goldsmith and Margolis (1979) found that dilatation and extraction (D&E) procedures for late terminations were more distressing for medical and nursing staff (because they often involve dismemberment of the fetus) than intra-amniotic methods. The opposite was the case for the women in this study however. Those who experienced labour and delivery of a dead fetus were more distressed by the procedure than those who experienced D&E.

## Psychological outcome of abortion

Do women experience depression, regret or traumatic reactions after abortion? It is in this area that most psychological research has concentrated and is least conclusive. Media evocations of a 'post abortion syndrome' have been hotly debated (Stotland, 1992), and the literature remains controversial although it has been thoroughly reviewed (e.g. Adler, David, Major et al., 1990; Zolese and Blacker, 1992; Turrell, Armsworth and Gaa, 1990; Posavac and Miller, 1990; Miller, 1992; etc.). Methodological problems are a major reason for the lack of conclusive findings (e.g. Wilmoth, de Alteriis and Bussell, 1992; Adler, David, Major et al., 1990; Turrell, Armsworth and Gaa, 1990; Zolese and Blacker, 1992). Potential respondents are often reluctant to participate or difficult to trace hence biasing the study sample. Control or comparison groups are difficult to identify, and the effects of abortion cannot be properly assessed without consideration of the effects of denied abortion, or the effects of full-term pregnancy. A wide variety of, often unstandardized, measures have been used to determine psychological outcomes (Posavac and Miller, 1990, found 112 dependent variable measures reported in the literature). Baseline psychological state before pregnancy is almost never assessed, (pre-abortion measures may themselves be influenced by the pregnancy or the impending procedure) and the timing of post-abortion assessment varies from 24 hours to several months. In addition, the field suffers from a failure to examine alternatives to the post-abortion trauma hypothesis, or develop predictive theories of psychological outcome (Posavac and Miller, 1990; Miller, 1992). Although this complex literature has been reviewed many times, the reviews themselves are often biased in their choice of studies to support either the 'post abortion syndrome' or 'no effect of abortion' depending upon the purpose of the authors (Wilmoth, de Alteriis and Bussell, 1992).

A useful statistical technique for combining a number of studies in a quantitative way, rather than a qualitative way as most literature reviews do, is meta-analysis. This technique has been used by Posavac and Miller (1990) for twenty-four studies which compared pre-abortion and post-abortion psychological states. The average effect size from this analysis was +0.606, hence overall women feel better after an abortion than before it. The average effect size for studies which compared women after an abortion with appropriate other groups was −0.086, hence women who have had an abortion are slightly worse off than women who haven't, but only by less than one-tenth of a standard deviation of the measures used. It should also be borne in mind that none of these studies incorporated pre-pregnancy measures, hence there is no way of knowing whether these groups differed before they became pregnant.

The studies included in this analysis were concerned with relatively short-term outcomes of abortion, and establish clearly that the situation and impending procedure are stressful for many women. The longer term outcomes are more difficult to assess because, as Wilmoth, de Alteriis and Bussell (1992) point out, women's lives are not static. A woman may feel better or worse a year after a termination than she did before but it is virtually impossible to know whether this is a consequence of the procedure or the many other events which will have occurred in the meantime. Gilligan and Belenky (1980) followed women for a year after an abortion decision was considered and found that for many of them the life crisis surrounding the abortion was associated with a shift to more mature and higher-level structures of thought. In other words, the resolution of the crisis had helped to move the women on to the next cognitive-developmental stage – a positive outcome, especially since many women cite their own psychological immaturity as a reason for having an abortion in the first place.

Zolese and Blacker (1992) reviewing the British literature on psychiatric consequences of abortion estimate that about 10 per cent of women will experience severe depression or anxiety in the year following a therapeutic abortion. The rates of psychiatric morbidity are higher amongst women whose desired pregnancy is terminated in the second trimester because of fetal abnormality or intra-uterine death (Iles and Gath, 1993).

These findings should of course be balanced against the psychological effects of denied abortion on both the mother and child. Dagg (1991) reviewing American studies of denied abortion showed that many women who are denied abortion continue to seek termination of their pregnancy, with about 40 per cent being successful. A higher than expected number of miscarriages (spontaneous abortions) are also reported. Women who carry their pregnancies to term are likely to keep the baby, with only about 11 per cent (average) being placed for adoption. The few studies which exist of these mothers and their children suggest that about one-third of the women experience guilt, anxiety and resentment of the child while the rest accept the child and are glad with hindsight that the pregnancy was not aborted (Pare and Raven, 1970). Being unwanted may also have a deleterious effect on the child (Forssman and Thuwe, 1966; Dagg, 1991).

Given that pregnancy termination can have negative effects for some women, two further questions arise. First, can we predict who will have a bad experience? And second, why is abortion a negative experience for some women? Recently some attempts have been made to address these questions. Turrell, Armsworth and Gaa (1990) found that women who were ambivalent about the abortion decision, or who felt that the decision was not their own (because of coercion by family, partner or professionals) were more likely to be distressed after the event. Other studies too have suggested that the degree of difficulty or ambivalence experienced in making the decision is associated with the degree of post-abortion distress (e.g. Adler, David, Major et al., 1990; Dagg, 1991; Cohan, Dunkel-Schetter and Lydon, 1993). Women whose pregnancy is being terminated for medical reasons have the highest rate of post-abortion distress (Iles and Gath, 1993; Illsey and Hall, 1976; Zolese and Blacker, 1992). Women with a previous psychiatric history (Dagg, 1991; Handy, 1982; Zolese and Blacker, 1992), and women who lack effective social support (Adler, David, Major et al., 1990; Zolese and Blacker, 1992) also fare less well than others.

Posavac and Miller (1990) propose five different hypotheses which may explain the positive psychological effects immediately after abortion:

1. **The relief hypothesis** suggests that pregnancy is a threat causing anxiety and stress which is relieved after the procedure.

2. **The dissonance hypothesis** suggests that a woman who has moral reservations about abortion but goes ahead anyway will relieve the cognitive dissonance by changing her attitudes towards abortion, and will thus feel better afterwards.
3. **The dissimulation hypothesis** suggests that women present themselves as psychologically distressed in order to obtain a termination and will therefore appear to be healthier afterwards as an artefact.
4. **The guilt hypothesis** explains the slight difference between women who have had an abortion and comparison groups as a result of the guilt some women feel from a morally controversial decision.
5. **The bonding hypothesis** suggests that women feel worse before the abortion than afterwards because of anticipatory grief.

These remain hypotheses, however, and require evaluation through carefully designed studies.

Miller (1992) identifies seven theoretical models implicit in the literature – two which are used to explain the short-term positive effects of abortion, and five which are used to explain the longer term negative effects. These models have not been tested explicitly by studies, but are implied by authors in their interpretation of results. The short-term positive effects are explained by a crisis model in which the anxiety created by an unwanted pregnancy is resolved by the abortion. Short-term negative effects are explained by a biological model which suggests that the physiological effects of pregnancy are interrupted by the abortion resulting in sudden and dramatic hormonal changes and transitory negative emotional states, similar to the 'baby blues' after childbirth.

The most common explanation for longer term effects is the stress model, which suggests that an unwanted pregnancy produces stress, this coupled with an abortion and a number of risk factors (e.g. inappropriate coping styles, lack of social support, previous mental illness, low self-esteem, etc.) can produce distress. Several other models are implied in the research literature. The norm violation model suggests that anti-abortion social norms produce conflict for a woman with an unwanted pregnancy, and result in guilt and shame if she goes through with it. The loss model suggests that women with an unwanted pregnancy vary in their desire to carry the pregnancy to term and experience loss and regret if the desire to continue the pregnancy is at odds with social or medical circumstances which advocate termination. This hypothesis can explain the negative outcomes if women feel coerced into a decision, or opt for a termination because of fetal abnormalities. The decision model suggests that the decision-making process before the abortion determines emotional states afterwards. If the effectiveness of the decision-making process was compromised because of situational, interpersonal or time constraints, negative feelings about the decision would be expected afterwards. The model also suggests that events after the abortion (e.g. an unsuccessful attempt to conceive) may cause negative feelings about the abortion decision. The learning model suggests that the unwanted pregnancy and abortion experience is a learning one for the woman. This may result in positive outcomes in terms of maturation and emotional development, or negative outcomes by creating fear and avoidance of sex, or disruption of existing relationships.

The data collected by Miller (1992) were used to test each of the models of long-term outcome, and the loss model was found to be the best predictor of regret. Some support was found for the other models, but ambivalence about the decision because of a woman's own childbearing desires or her perceived coercion to have an abortion were by far the best predictors of longer term regret and distress. As Miller points out, his study was not designed to test each of these models thoroughly and further research is needed, but this analysis does reinforce the need for good theoretically derived studies in this area.

## Conclusions

Abortion is an emotive topic which has moral and physical aspects as well as psychological ones. The research in this field has been influenced by political and moral debates so that the questions asked by psychologists have tended to reflect the assumptions inherent in contemporary western thinking about abortion, rather than the actual experience. Hence, most of the research has investigated the supposed difficulty of the decision-making process and the presumed negative psychological outcomes of abortion. This research has shown that for most women the decision to have an abortion is made very quickly (even before she knows that she is pregnant), and the psychological outcomes are minimal. Amongst women who do have difficulty making the decision, regret and depression are more likely, but for some women the resolution of the dilemma has positive psychological consequences resulting in increased emotional maturity. The research has been fraught with methodological difficulties and, until recently, largely lacking in explicit theoretical models. However, some practical implications can be derived in terms of counselling women who request abortions.

Psychological research on abortion has largely been concerned with the assessment of common-sense notions of it. Hence, the idea that some women are more likely to terminate their pregnancies than others, and the investigation of post-abortion trauma. There have been very few studies which begin from a description of women's experiences as described by themselves and which develop theories inductively rather than deductively. This type of research is badly needed if the purpose of psychology is to understand how women and their clinicians decide on abortion and how they cope with the decision.

## Applications

### 1. Abortion counselling

Women who experience ambivalence in making the abortion decision, or who feel that the decision is not their own, experience more post-abortion regret and distress than those who do not. Counsellors then need to help women to explore their own feelings independently of their family members and facilitate the decision-making process, so that, whichever decision a woman makes, she feels that it is her own decision.

The approach to counselling needs to take into account the emotional development of the woman concerned and stage of the decision-making process which she has reached. Many women will have completed this process before they encounter medical professionals and will not need in-depth counselling. Those concerned must be sensitive to the individual needs of each woman and avoid stereotyping abortion seekers.

### 2. The abortion procedure

The abortion procedure is stressful for clients and for staff, especially in the case of late abortions. Techniques for reducing patient anxiety around other medical procedures could be applied to abortion clients. For example, clear information about the procedure should be provided, and the process should be explained at each step. Staff stress may be reduced by use of support groups.

## Further reading

Wilmoth, G. (ed). (1992). Psychological Perspectives on Abortion and Its Alternatives. Special issue of the *Journal of Social Issues*, **48**, No. 3.

## References

Adler, N., David, H., Major, B., Roth, S., Russo, N. and Wyatt, G. (1990). Psychological responses after abortion. *Science*, **248**, 41–4.

Allen, I. (1981). *Family Planning, Abortion and Sterilisation Services*. No. 595. London: The Policy Studies Institute.

Baetson, K., Rankin, R., Fuller, G. et al. (1985). A comparative MMPI study of abortion seeking women and those who intend to carry their pregnancies to term. *Family Practice Research Journal*, **4**, 199–207.

Beard, R., Belsey, E., Lai, S., Lewis, S. and Greer, H. (1974). King's Termination Study II: Contraceptive practice before and after outpatient termination of pregnancy. *British Medical Journal*, 1, 418–21.

Boyle, M. (1991). Decision making for contraception and abortion. In *The Psychology of Health: An Introduction*. (M. Pitts and K. Phillips, eds) pp. 156–70. London: Routledge.

Boyle, M. (1992). The abortion debate: an analysis of psychological assumptions underlying legislation and professional decision-making. In *The Psychology of Women's Health and Health Care* (P. Nicholson and J. Ussher, eds) pp. 124–51. London: Macmillan.

Boyle, M. (1993). The abortion debate: A neglected issue in psychology? *The Psychologist: Bulletin of the British Psychological Society*, 6, 106–9.

Bracken, M., Klerman, L. and Bracken, M. (1978a). Coping with pregnancy resolution among never-married women. *American Journal of Orthopsychiatry*, 48, 320–34.

Bracken, M., Klerman, L. and Bracken, M. (1978b). Abortion, adoption or motherhood: An empirical study of decision-making during pregnancy. *American Journal of Obstetrics and Gynaecology*, 130, 251–62.

Broome, A. (1984). Termination of pregnancy. In *Psychology and Gynaecological Problems* (A. Broome and L. Wallace, eds) pp. 60–76. London: Tavistock.

Cohan, C., Dunkel-Schetter, C. and Lydon, J. (1993). Pregnancy decision making: Predictors of early stress and adjustment. *Psychology of Women Quarterly*, 17, 223–40.

Coote, A., Harman, H. and Hewitt, P. (1990). *The Family Way*. Social Policy Paper No. 1, London: Institute for Public Policy Research.

Costa, F., Jessor, R. and Donovan, J. (1987). Psychosocial correlates and antecedents of abortion: An exploratory study. *Population and Environment*, 9, 3–22.

Dagg, P. (1991). The psychological sequelae of therapeutic abortion – denied and completed. *American Journal of Psychiatry*, 148, 578–85.

Fishbein, M. and Ajzen, I. (1975). *Belief, Attitude, Intention and Behaviour: An Introduction to Theory and Research*. Reading, MA: Addison-Wesley.

Fiske, S. and Taylor, S. (1991). *Social Cognition*. 2nd edn. New York: McGraw Hill.

Ford, C., Castelnuovo-Tedesco, P. and Long, K. (1972). Women who seek therapeutic abortion compared with women completing pregnancy. *American Journal of Psychiatry*, 129, 546–52.

Forssman, H. and Thuwe, I. (1966). One hundred and twenty children born after application for therapeutic abortion refused. *Acta Psychiatrica Scandinavica*, 42, 71–8.

Gilligan, C. (1982). *In A Different Voice: Psychological Theory and Women's Development*. Cambridge, MA: Harvard University Press.

Gilligan, C. and Belenky, M. (1980). A naturalistic study of abortion decisions. In *Clinical-Developmental Psychology* (R. Selman and R. Yando, eds) pp. 69–90. New Directions for Child Development, No. 7. San Francisco: Jossey-Bass.

Green, J., Snowdon, C. and Statham, H. (1993). Pregnant women's attitudes to abortion and prenatal screening. *Journal of Reproductive and Infant Psychology*, 11, 31–9.

Hamill, E. and Ingram, I. (1974). Psychiatric factors in the abortion decision. *British Medical Journal*, i, 229–32.

Handy, J. (1982). Psychological and social aspects of induced abortion. *British Journal of Clinical Psychology*, 21, 29–41.

Humphries, S. (1988). *A Secret World of Sex. Forbidden Fruit: The British Experience: 1900–1950*. London: Sidgwick and Jackson.

Iles, S. and Gath, D. (1993). Psychiatric outcome of termination of pregnancy for foetal abnormality. *Psychological Medicine*, 23, 407–13.

Illsey, R. and Hall, H. (1976). Psychosocial aspects of abortion: A review of issues and needed research. *Bulletin of the World Health Organisation*, 53, 83–106.

Kaltreider, N., Goldsmith, S. and Margolis, A. (1979). The impact of mid-trimester abortion techniques on patients and staff. *American Journal of Obstetrics and Gynaecology*, 135, 235–8.

Luker, K. (1984). The war between the women. *Family Planning Perspectives*, 16, 105–10.

Miller, W. (1992). An empirical study of the psychological antecedents and consequences of induced abortion. *Journal of Social Issues*, 48, 67–94.

Osofsky, J. and Osofsky, H. (1972). The psychological reactions of patients to legalized abortions. *American Journal of Orthopsychiatry*, **42**, 48–59.

Pare, C. and Raven, H. (1970). Psychiatric sequelae to therapeutic abortion: follow-up of patients referred for termination of pregnancy. *Lancet*, **1**, 635–8.

Phoenix, A. (1991). *Young Mothers?* Oxford: Polity.

Pipes, M. (1986). *Understanding Abortion*. London: The Women's Press.

Posavac, E. and Miller, T. (1990). Some problems caused by not having a conceptual foundation for health research: An illustration from studies of the psychological effects of abortion. *Psychology and Health*, **5**, 13–23.

Rafferty, P. (1993). Psychological intervention with gynaecological surgery patients. *Journal of Reproductive and Infant Psychology*, **11**, 1, Supplement 1 (Conference Abstracts) p. 6.

Russo, N., Horn, J. and Schwartz, R. (1992). U.S. abortion in context: Selected characteristics and motivations of women seeking abortions. *Journal of Social Issues*, **48**, 183–202.

Shorter, E. (1983). *A History of Women's Bodies*. London: Allen Lane.

Simms, M. (1974). Midwives and abortion in the 1930s. *Midwife and Health Visitor*, **10**, 115.

Slade, P. (1994) Predicting the psychological impact of miscarriage. *Journal of Reproductive and Infant Psychology*, **12**, 5–16.

Smetana, J. and Adler, N. (1979). Decision-making regarding abortion: A value x expectancy analysis. *Journal of Population*, **2**, 348–55.

Smith, T. (1993). Influence of socioeconomic factors on attaining targets for reducing teenage pregnancies. *British Medical Journal*, **306**, 1232–5.

Stotland, N. (1992). The myth of the abortion trauma syndrome. *Journal of the American Medical Association*, **268**, 2078–9.

Tew, M. (1990). *Safer Childbirth? A Critical History of Maternity Care*. London: Chapman and Hall.

Torres, A. and Forest, J. (1988). Why do women have abortions? *Family Planning Perspectives*, **20**, 169–76.

Turrell, S., Armsworth, M. and Gaa, J. (1990). Emotional response to abortion: a critical review of the literature. *Women and Therapy*, **9**, 49–68.

Vayreda, A. and Antaki, C. (1991). Explanations in abortion discourses. *Text*, **11**, 481–98.

Williams, J. (1987). *Psychology of Women: Behaviour in a Biosocial Context*. 3rd edn. New York: W. W. Norton.

Wilmoth, G., de Alteriis, M. and Bussell, D. (1992). Prevalence of psychological risks following legal abortion in the U.S.: Limits of the evidence. *Journal of Social Issues*, **48**, 37–66.

Zolese, G. and Blacker, C. (1992). The psychological complications of therapeutic abortion. *British Journal of Psychiatry*, **160**, 742–9.

# Psychological aspects of sexual behaviour and HIV disease[1]

## Lorraine Sherr

> No book on reproduction would be complete without some discussion of sexual behaviour and sexuality and these are the topics covered in the final two chapters. A major influence both on sexual behaviour and research in this field in recent years has been the spread of HIV and AIDS. There can be few people who are now unaware of the existence of HIV and its relationship to the fatal disease AIDS. In the absence of any medical cure for the disease, the only hope for limiting its spread lies in prevention of infection. This requires people to make changes to their sexual behaviour and habits. In this chapter Lorraine Sherr explores the contribution which psychology has made to an understanding of who will practise 'safe sex' and when. Do frightening advertising campaigns change people's behaviour? Can beliefs and attitudes predict condom use? Does counselling reduce HIV transmission?

## Introduction

Human Immunodeficiency Virus (HIV) is essentially a sexually transmitted disease which has emerged in the latter part of this century. It is associated with Acquired Immune Deficiency Syndrome (AIDS) which compromises immune functioning leading to a wide range of opportunistic infections and ultimately death. Infection can also occur transplacentally and through blood and body fluids. Infection is life-long and, despite many medical advances in treatment and management, the only effective tool against transmission is prevention of initial exposure. Essentially this is achieved through behavioural change, especially through changes in sexual behaviour. The emergence of the HIV and AIDS pandemic has widespread implications for sexual expression, relationships, education, reproduction and medical care.

A diagnosis of HIV infection has profound and life-long ramifications on an individual. There is a high psychological morbidity associated with HIV infection (Ostrow, 1990). Indeed, even entering the testing process itself may be associated with emotional trauma, irrespective of test outcome. Life may be severely challenged in the presence of HIV infection. Individuals have to cope not only with possible disease and death, but with a wide range of oscillating emotions triggered by isolation, anxiety, social stigma, sexuality questions, reproduction issues, uncertainty, economic and social hardship, possible ill health and dependency (Miller, 1990).

Early research on AIDS prevention and management set the agenda. It was thought that the message was simple. If individuals refrained from sex or maintained monogamy between uninfected partners and always used condoms with new partners transmission would be curtailed. Not so. Such a simplistic solution reflects little understanding of human behaviour, relationships, prompts, triggers,

[1] Copyright Lorraine Sherr

negotiation skills, roles and power balances let alone the ability to sustain these over time and within varying situations.

## HIV/AIDS and sexual behaviour

Research into AIDS prevention has examined sexual behaviour and behaviour change in a number of contexts. Firstly researchers have investigated general population behaviour in the light of HIV infection. Secondly, specific behaviours associated with those who, through their behaviour or social grouping, may be at a heightened risk of exposure to HIV infection, have been studied. Lastly, studies have considered the group who are already infected and whose behaviour adjustment may curtail further spread of the infection.

The HIV epidemic has highlighted how little is known about sexual behaviour. Sexual behaviour in context must be understood if there is to be any progress towards understanding behaviour change. Factors which may contribute to such an understanding include age, relationship style (e.g. casual or regular), sexual orientation (e.g. heterosexual, homosexual), gender, the context of sexual behaviour (e.g. commercial sex, alcohol or drug associated), reproduction issues, contraception issues and normative pressures (e.g. peer group or societal influences). Sexual behaviour cannot be viewed in isolation from gender roles (Wight, 1990; Holland, 1991). This may mean that partners within a relationship perceive different roles for themselves and attribute responsibility for safer sex to the other person. It is presumptuous to think that all sexual encounters are equal and that dialogue is always possible. In situations of rape, abuse and intimidation this would not be so. In commercial sex the roles are also complex.

Wight (1990) notes a reluctance to talk about sexual behaviour which results in limited insight into the sexual history of partners and may impede any dialogue or negotiation of safer sexual practices between them. Ingham, Woodcock and Stenner (1991) elaborate on this silence and failure to engage in dialogue. They maintain that if a partner is willing to reveal previous sexual history this very act may jeopardize any trust or belief in confidentiality. Holland, Ramazanoglu, Scott et al. (1991) also note that any sexual history dialogue which can infer suspicion has relationship implications.

## Women and HIV/AIDS

Research about HIV/AIDS among women is sparse (Sherr and Strong, 1991; Holland, Ramazanoglu, Scott et al., 1992). Globally, there are more men with HIV than women. However, female to male transmission is less efficient than male to female transmission (van de Wijgert and Padian, 1993), and the risk of becoming infected from a one-off heterosexual contact is twice to twenty times less likely from woman to man than vice versa (Padian, Shiboski and Jewell, 1991; Rehmet, Staszewski, Muller et al., 1992). Thus, currently women are at a greater risk of infection.

Few studies examine the extent to which behaviour change is feasible for women and which means are used by women to accomplish this (Richardson, 1990). Worth (1990) notes that the most common response to risk of infection for a woman is not the use of condoms in her sexual encounters but restriction to one partner, altering partners or having less sex (Wofsy, 1988). Yet such behaviour may still expose women to risk if their sexual partners share needles, have multiple partners themselves or are in the sex industry (Worth, 1990; Wofsy,

1988; Piot, Plummer and Rey, 1987; Ngugi, Plummer and Simonsen, 1988; Williams, Hearst and Udofia et al., 1989; Wilson, Chiroro, Lavelle and Mutero, 1989; Day, Ward and Harris, 1988; Mann, Nzilambi and Piot, 1988). Women who suggest alternatives to penetrative sex may endanger their relationships and the self-esteem of their male partners.

Many studies fail to recognize that sexual decision making for women is not straightforward (Sherr and Strong, 1991). It may not simply be knowledge that engenders behaviour change, but more complex notions concerned with socio-economic standing, power, self-esteem, dependency, culture and the competing challenges of a desire to conceive and the desire to protect themselves (Sherr, 1993a).

### HIV/AIDS and pregnancy

HIV infection in women can either be established prior to pregnancy, or high-lighted during routine ante-natal care (Sherr, 1993b). In the UK, Davison, Holland, Newell et al., (1993) note that of known HIV-positive pregnant women, one-third were first identified at ante-natal clinics in England, Wales and Northern Ireland. This figure was as high as 59 per cent for the Irish Republic. Yet few ante-natal clinics discuss sexual behaviour or condom use.

One of the major issues raised is the possibility of termination of pregnancy in the presence of HIV infection. Termination of pregnancy is a procedure which should never be taken lightly, as it may have long-term psychological ramifications for all concerned (Sherr, 1993b). Although the offer of termination is often put forward as the reason for screening in the first place, uptake of screening and termination in the presence of HIV is often low (Johnston, Brettle, MacCallum et al., 1989; Stratton, 1990; Sunderland, Minkoff, Handte et al., 1992; Selwyn, Carter and Schoenbaum, 1989). Furthermore, those who do opt for termination may well proceed to a subsequent pregnancy, irrespective of HIV factors (Sunderland, Minkoff, Handte et al., 1992). There are no studies which examine the psychological costs or benefits to women of termination of pregnancy in the presence of HIV infection. From the general literature it is clear that short-term trauma can be anticipated, but long-term adjustment is usually good. With HIV the termination may be inextricably bound with the infection and the longer term ramifications may be less positive.

There are reported positive emotions associated with pregnancy in the presence of HIV infection. Mothers with an HIV-positive child are willing to consider a subsequent pregnancy (Temmerman, Mosses, Kiragu et al., 1990), and those who have children report many positive aspects associated with the fulfilment of parenting, the joy of the children and the added meaning it may give to their lives. Personal dilemmas about parenting can be fraught (Levine and Dubler, 1990) and decision making may be linked to optimism especially when associated with prior knowledge of a baby born virus-free (Kurth and Hutchinson, 1990).

## Psychological approaches to HIV/AIDS prevention

The onset of the HIV/AIDS epidemic prompted worldwide preventive initiatives. Many of these were based on the assumption that knowledge alone would alter behaviour, with scant attention being paid to the vast body of theoretical literature which explores the complexity of human behaviour, decision making and attitude formation.

Information is paramount in order that any individual can understand the potential threat posed by HIV and identify individual behavioural patterns or acts that may be classified as 'risky'. Such information may be a necessary ingredient in the process of change, but does not suffice as the only ingredient prompting wholesale change. Studies have shown that knowledge about AIDS may not even be a predictor of change. Di Clemente, Forrest and Micker (1990) found a negative correlation between levels of knowledge and behaviour change, whilst Ross and Kelahar (1993) comment that perceived personal susceptibility may be more important as a predictor of behaviour change than knowledge. Studies such as these are difficult to interpret, however, because they correlate individual knowledge with behaviour which essentially occurs within a couple. This does not reflect the combination of knowledge, knowledge sharing (if it occurs), and conflicting knowledge within a couple, or the influence of inter-personal and situational dynamics on behaviour.

Preventive behaviour initiatives have centred around encouraging individuals to use condoms, reduce numbers of sexual partners, and to avoid anal inter-course. A growing body of literature suggests, however, that sexual behaviour is extremely difficult to manipulate or change (Sherr, 1987; Hart, 1989; Kelly, Lawrence, Hood and Brasfield, 1989). In addition, most studies of preventive behaviour are cross-sectional in nature and do not give a comprehensive longer term insight. Longitudinal studies have found that sexual behaviour change is very difficult to sustain (Joseph, Montgomer, Kessler et al., 1988: McCusker, Stoddard, McDonald et al., 1992; Kelly, St Lawrence and Brasfield, 1991; Ekstrand, 1992).

## Knowledge, attitude and behaviour studies

Many of the 'knowledge, attitude and behaviour' studies spawned in the wake of the AIDS epidemic (Ross and Kelaher, 1993) have been of limited utility given their scant attention to theory. In general, population type studies have utilized similar methodologies and there are a number of common themes in their findings. The studies comprise a mixture of information measures (questions about HIV/AIDS which assess the individual's attitudes and level of knowledge) and reports of sexual behaviour. They are either conducted by telephone inter-view, face-to-face interview or through anonymous questionnaires (Hingson, Strunin, Carven et al., 1989; Sherr, Strong and Goldmeier, 1990; Hooykas, van der Linden, van Doornam et al., 1991). Given that sexual behaviour is the major outcome variable there are enormous constraints on such findings. Self-reports may suffer from a number of biases. Individual may report socially acceptable rather than accurate personal data or they may have limited recall. There are few studies which have attempted to check such outcomes. Some studies have used the presence of other sexually transmitted diseases as an outcome index (Plummer, Moses, Jackoniah and Ndinya Achola, 1991). This has clear utility, but may be limited in application to non-STD sufferers. Some studies have compared partners' reports of sexual activity (e.g. Wilson, 1993) often finding high levels of agreement.

Few studies have utilized standard information measures. Many include elements of knowledge on transmission and risk. Yet others question respondents on epidemiology and causal transmission. It is unclear to what extent accurate knowledge of these questions may relate to sexual behaviour and whether they should be given equal weighting in any composite knowledge 'score'. Most studies generate their own idiosyncratic knowledge items and behaviour measures, thus rendering comparisons very difficult.

Di Clemente, Forrest and Micker (1990) surveyed 1127 adolescents in the USA and found that despite sound levels of information regarding risks of HIV transmission, multiple sexual partners were commonly recorded and condom use was particularly low (only 8 per cent consistently using them). Sherr, Strong and Goldmeier (1990) examined condom use and sexual behaviour in a sample of 260 STD clinic attenders. They found risky behaviour prevalent. The only predictor of unsafe sex was 'the actual desire for unprotected sex'. Furthermore there was no relationship between current condom use and the recognition, endorsement or influence of UK health education material.

Uitenbrook and McQueen (1992) surveyed 9416 Scottish respondents (aged 18 to 44) to explore the link between HIV knowledge and risky behaviours. They found behavioural change both in terms of partner number and condom usage. This varied according to gender and educational level.

## Intervention studies

Intervention studies have often reported behaviour change, yet the mechanisms of such change are unclear. For example, Walter and Vaughan (1992) compared reported knowledge, behaviours, beliefs and self-efficacy in a group of 1316 high school students randomly allocated to an intervention group or control group. They found some evidence of behaviour change sustained at three months.

Two main problems arise when evaluating behaviour change, however. First, total behaviour change is required to eradicate new infections, but partial behaviour change is often reported (Stall, Coates and Hoff, 1989; Becker and Joseph, 1988; McCusick, Coates, Morin et al., 1990; Ekstrand and Coates, 1990). For example, Di Clemente, Forrest and Micker (1990) showed that one in three of their respondents reported some form of behaviour change. Thus both new infection and behaviour change are possible. Second, the initial adoption of a new behaviour is easier than long-term maintenance. This has been shown in areas of smoking research (Sutton and Eiser, 1984; Warner, 1981), alcohol consumption (Kleinot and Rogers, 1982), dietary studies and seat belt utiliz-ation (Sutton and Eiser, 1990). Such findings may account for the low and fluctuating levels of maintenance of safe sex found within large cohorts studies over time. For example, Beltran, Ostrow and Joseph (1993) examined factors associated with sexual behaviour change in a longitudinal cohort study. Those who reported an 'adverse sexual behaviour change' had reported (prior to HIV testing), higher levels of mental distress, denial, fatalism, coping strategies and low levels of social support.

Fear arousal was the option most utilized in early HIV and AIDS campaigns as the means to accomplish behaviour change. Scant attention was paid to the vast body of literature which points to the limitations of fear arousal as a prompt for behaviour change (Leventhal, 1970). It is unclear why such fear arousal tactics are ineffective, although there are several possible explanations. It may be that the emotional load is such that subjects deny the threat. Alternatively, it may be that fear-arousing messages do not frighten the subjects. The recommended action may not be perceived to be effective (Sutton, 1982), or it may be that cognitive factors are related to behavioural intention independently of fear

(Sutton, in press). Two opposing theories need to be examined if light is to be shed on the disparate findings. They both examine the relationship between fear and behaviour change but conclude an 'inverted U' relationship on the one hand compared to a linear relationship on the other. Janis (1967) describes a relationship between fear and behaviour change as one of an inverted U. Linear theories would predict highest efficacy for high-fear appeals, where inverted U theories would predict limited or zero effect for high-fear situations. Sherr (1990) showed that HIV fear arousing campaigns targeted at drug users did not raise anxiety levels and were ineffective in reported behaviour change. However, they did have an anxiety effect on non-target groups. Sherr (1994) also noted that humour was more likely to be recognized, endorsed and promote influence than fear-arousing death images.

### Relationship factors

Sexual behaviour studies may be limited when they do not include the context of relationships. General findings have shown that for many groups condom use is more likely with casual partners than with regular partners. Often the closeness of a relationship can directly affect condom uptake or continuation (Donoghoe, Stimson, Dolan and Alldritt, 1989). Many studies now examine behaviour change in terms of factors such as negotiation, power, disclosure, lies, trust and convenience. These give insight into the complex nature of human interactions. Studies have shown that partner disclosure may not occur (Manoloto, Hayes and Padre, 1990), especially if there is no other means of survival. Indeed other studies have documented that partners would lie about their HIV status (Cochran and Mays, 1990) on the one hand, or be unable to discuss HIV on the other (Wilkins, Alonso, Baldeh et al., 1989).

### Theoretical contributions

Few studies have attempted to turn to theory to shed light on the complexity of sexual behaviour, risk behaviour and behaviour change. The most promising insights emerge when this is done.

Overviews of the wide range of studies have consistently concluded that knowledge levels have a limited effect on behaviour change (Ross and Kelaher, 1993). This could be accounted for by ceiling effects in the worldwide dissemination of basic AIDS knowledge, or by more complex variables which intervene between knowledge and behaviour. Psychological theory has driven a number of studies to elaborate on these factors and these studies serve to explain behavioural factors and also may give direction to future interventions.

Weinstein (1988) proposes a model of 'precaution adoption'. This model as applied to HIV/AIDS suggests that people progress from an initial stage of unawareness about the condition to a stage of awareness and an understanding that HIV/AIDS has implications for them. After this stage they may progress to a stage of decision making about their own behaviour, followed by a stage of action planning. Only after progression through all of these stages will action actually be taken to change behaviour. According to this model, an input of knowledge would raise awareness and feed into decision making but not contribute much further.

Health belief models (e.g. Becker, 1974) may shed light on the barriers to behavioural change (Johnson, Ostrow and Joseph, 1990). These theories allow for the incorporation of motivation, personal risk perceptions, social norms and allied intentions. Generally they propose that factors associated with behaviour change include knowledge about the condition, perception of personal risk, belief that behaviour change can reduce risk, behavioural intentions and social norm influences. Other theories which have been applied to behaviour change in the context of HIV/AIDS are Fishbein and Ajzen's (1975) theory of reasoned action (TRA) and Bandura's social learning theory (SLT – Bandura, 1984). TRA suggests that perceptions of preference may influence the adoption of a new behaviour, while SLT introduces the influence of social reinforcement.

Such models have elaborated on the cognitive processes associated with behavioural change (Emmons, Joseph and Kessler, 1986). Strunin and Hingson (1993) examined adolescent behaviour according to the health belief model and found that respondents who believed condoms were effective in HIV prevention and who were also worried about perceived vulnerability to AIDS were 3.1 times more likely to report consistent condom use than were respondents who carried condoms and had discussed their use with their doctor. Allard (1989) showed that beliefs about AIDS could affect sexual risk taking and condom use.

Weinstein (1983) has shown that individuals invoke an 'optimistic bias' about their own health vulnerability. Both personal and response efficacy must be high to prompt behaviour change. If individuals believe they are able to effect change and that change is effective in reducing risk, they are more likely to change their behaviour than if they do not believe this (McCusick, Wiley and Coates, 1985). Even when individuals know about potential risks associated with their behaviour, difficulties with sexual impulse control may be an overriding factor (Johnson, Ostrow and Joseph, 1990).

Cognitive beliefs appear to contribute to change in behaviour but cannot account for all the reported change (Friedman, Des Jarlais, Ward et al., 1993). Normative influences (Abdul Quader, Tross and Friedman, 1990), peer group influences (Friedman et al., 1993; Coutinho, van Griensven and Moss, 1989), coping (Martin, 1993; Perkins, Leserman, Murphy and Evans, 1993) and contextual factors are also important.

For example, in an in-depth study of 340 subjects, Gold, Karmiloff Smith, Skinner and Morton (1992) investigated the justifications given for 'unsafe' sexual encounters. These included the use of alternative contraception (which would be effective against pregnancy but not prophylactic to HIV), perceived low risk of heterosexuals, beliefs about the partner based on observable characteristics (e.g. intelligence, appearance, educational level), use of alcohol, condom availability and boredom. Similarly, Keller (1993) found a high rate of unsafe encounters, often triggered by the spontaneity of the event or on partner judgements based on appearance or intuition alone in a study of 272 students.

Models which explore the nature of behaviour in context hold out more hope for future health intervention initiatives than those focusing solely on cognitions.

## Links between attitude and behaviour change

Generally studies have shown that no single psychological theory can be utilized to explain risky sexual behaviour or guarantee behaviour change. An integration of a number of theoretical elements may be the way forward. Chapman, Stoker,

Ward et al. (1990) examined the relationship between attitudes and beliefs about condoms and protective behaviour in 408 sexually active young adults. They explored specific attitudes to condoms and found that those who found condom use embarrassing and incompatible with good sex were more likely to be irregular or non-users of condoms. They also found that perceived personal susceptibility to AIDS was different from other sexually transmitted diseases. Those who had self-perceptions of susceptibility to the former were more likely to use condoms. Lupton (1992) on the other hand, was unable to establish a link between positive attitudes towards condom use and consistent condom use during sex.

Basen Engquist (1992) studied 275 university students to examine condom use and AIDS related dialogue within sexual couples. Basen Engquist noted that coping style (information avoiding), perceived barriers and perceived susceptibility were significant predictors of intention to use condoms. This study also found that high self-efficacy and strong social support predicted the intention to discuss AIDS and previous sexual history with a new partner. The most important finding from this study is the independence of these two intentions. It seems that intention to use condoms and intention to discuss AIDS are not related to each other.

These studies emphasize the links between attitudes and behaviour change but also identify other crucial factors, such as social skills (Treffke, Tiggerman and Ross, 1992). Clearly explanations of behaviour and attempts to change behaviour must consider the context of the individual and the sexual activity as well as her or his attitudes and beliefs.

## Counselling and behaviour change

The role of counselling in HIV/AIDS related behaviour change has not been systematically evaluated. Mass media and educational efforts were not the only source of AIDS and HIV related information and potential triggers of behaviour change. The introduction of an HIV test prompted widespread counselling, particularly surrounding testing. Although it was not made explicit that one of the roles of such counselling would be to promote behavioural change, such change was often employed as an outcome measure, indeed as an index of efficacy at times. Higgins, Galavotti, O'Reilly et al., (1991) provided a comprehensive review of counselling, testing and behaviour studies. These included studies of homosexual men, intravenous drug users, pregnant women and 'other heterosexuals'. One of the problems highlighted by this review is the blurring of outcome measures. For example, among gay men outcome measures included reductions in anal sex, use of condoms and a reduction in the number of partners, while among pregnant women, termination of pregnancy was the main outcome measure for nearly all of the studies (Higgins, Galavotti, O'Reilly et al., 1991). None looked at sexual behaviour in pregnant women, despite the fact that current evidence suggests that having multiple sexual partners during pregnancy may increase the risk of vertical transmission.

In general, such overviews highlight the limitations of one-off counselling sessions. They also point out the difficulty of measuring behavioural change as an outcome of counselling when this may not have been the reason for counselling in the first place. Counselling in the presence of HIV may result in different outcomes. Padian, O'Brien, Chang et al. (1993) followed 144 couples from 1985 who received couple counselling and risk assessment regularly at six-monthly intervals. They found significant increases in condom use and sexual abstinence over time. The most dramatic behaviour change occurred on entry into the project, and no seroconversions in the HIV negative partner were observed for this study, accounting for '193 couple years'. Yet risk exposure was noted in a study by Kennedy, Skurnick, Wan et al., (1993) in an analysis of 106 sexually active couples, one of whom was HIV positive in each case. This study noted gender effects in relation to condom use as well as alcohol and drug effects. No record of seroconversions were taken in this study.

In general such studies have shown that limited behaviour change is consistently reported, but total change is rare (Higgins, Galavotti, O'Reilly et al., 1991). Behaviour change can encompass both sexual and drug using behaviour (Friedman, Des Jarlais, Ward et al., 1993) and there is often a link between these (Abdul Quader, Tross and Friedman, 1990).

## Conclusion

HIV and AIDS have brought a new facet to sexual expression which cannot be overlooked. Years of health and sex education can be undermined by the misuse of fear-associated images linking love and sex with death. Yet there is a challenge to health educators to understand sexual behaviour and to create an environment where protection from HIV infection is endorsed. Psychological theory that attempts to highlight sexual behaviour needs to take on board the complexities of such human interaction.

Acknowledgement to the EC project on Ante Natal HIV testing.

---

## Applications

### 1. Information about HIV/AIDS
Frightening advertising campaigns are unlikely to encourage people to change their sexual behaviours. However, good quality, accurate and detailed information is needed about HIV/AIDS and 'risky' behaviours as a first step towards behaviour change.

### 2. Putting behaviour in context
Attitudes and beliefs about HIV/AIDS and condom use are important, but often not enough to predict 'risky' activities. Health educators need to focus on the context of sexual behaviour and the development of assertiveness and negotiation skills in sexual encounters if condoms are to be used reliably.

# Further reading

Aggleton, P., Davies, P. and Hart, G. (eds) (1991). *AIDS Responses: Intervention and Care*. Brighton: Falmer Press.
Ostrow, D. (ed.) (1990). *Behavioural Aspects of AIDS*. New York: Plenum Press.
Sherr, L. (1991). *HIV and AIDS in Mothers and Babies*. Oxford: Blackwell Scientific Publications.
Squire, C. (ed.) (1993). *AIDS and Women*. London: Sage.

# References

Abdul Quader, A., Tross, S. and Friedman, S. (1990). Street recruited iv drug users and sexual risk reduction in New York City. *AIDS*, **4**, 1075–9.
Allard, R. (1989). Beliefs about AIDS as determinants of preventive practices and support for coercive measures. *American Journal of Public Health*, **79**, 448–52.
Aral, S., Cates, W. and Jenkins, W. (1985). Does knowledge lead to action? *American Journal of Public Health*, **75**, 69–71.
Bandura, A. (1984). Self efficacy: Toward a unifying theory of behavioural change. *Psychological Review*, **84**, 191–215.
Basen Engquist, K. (1992). Psychosocial predictors of safer sex behaviours in young adults. *AIDS Education and Prevention*, **4**, 120–34.
Becker, M. (1974). *The Health Belief Model Thorofare*. New Jersey: Slack.
Becker, M. and Joseph, J. (1988). AIDS and behavioral change to reduce risk a review. *American Journal of Public Health*, **78**, 394–410.
Beltran, E., Ostrow, D. and Joseph, J. (1993). Predictors of sexual behavior change among men requesting their HIV 1 antibody status. *AIDS Education and Prevention*, **5**, 3, 185–95.
Chapman, S., Stoker, L., Ward, M., Porritt, D. and Fahey, P. (1990). Discriminant attitudes and beliefs about condoms in young multi partner heterosexuals. *International Journal of STD and AIDS*, **1**, 422–8.
Cochran, S. and Mays, V. (1990). Sex, lies and HIV. *New England Journal of Medicine*, **322**, 774–5.
Coutinho, R., van Griensven, G. and Moss, A. (1989). Effects of preventive efforts among homosexual men. *AIDS*, **3**, sup. 1, p. s53–6.
Davison, C., Holland, F. Newell, M., Hudson, C. and Peckham, C. (1993). Screening for HIV infection in pregnancy. *AIDS Care*, **5**, 2, 135–40.
Day, S., Ward, H. and Harris, J. R. W. (1988). Prostitute women and public health. *British Medical Journal*, **297**, 1585.
Di Clemente, R., Forrest, K., and Micker, S. (1990). College students' knowledge and attitudes about AIDS and changes in HIV preventive behaviours. *AIDS Education and Prevention*, **2**, 201–12.
Donoge, M., Stimson, G., Dolan, K. and Alldritt, L. L. (1989). Sexual behaviour of injecting drug users and associated risks of HIV infection for non injecting partners. *AIDS Care*, **1**, 103–9.
Eckstrand, M. (1992). Safer sex maintenance among gay men: are we making any progress? *AIDS*, **6**, 875–7.
Eckstrand, M. and Coates, T. (1990). Maintenance of safer sexual behavior and predictors of risky sex: The San Francisco Men's Health Study. *American Journal of Public Health*, **80**, 973–7.
Emmons, C., Joseph, J. and Kessler, R. (1986). Psychosocial predictors of reported behavior change in homosexual men at risk for AIDS. *Health Education Quarterly*, **13**, 331–45.
Fishbein, M. and Ajzen, I. (1975). *Belief, Attitude, Intention and Behaviour: An Introduction to Theory and Research*. Reading, MA; Addison Wesley.
Friedman, S., Des Jarlais, D., Ward, T., Jose, B., Neaigus, A. and Goldstein, M. (1993). Drug injectors and heterosexual AIDS. In *AIDS in the Heterosexual Population* (L. Sherr, ed.). Switzerland: Harwood Academic.
Gold, R., Karmiloff, Smith, A., Skinner, M. and Morton, J. (1992). Situational factors and thought processes associated with unprotected intercourse in heterosexual students. *AIDS Care*, **4**, 3, 305–23.
Hart, G. (1989). Injecting drug use, HIV and AIDS editorial. *AIDS Care*, **1**, 3, 237–45.

Higgins, D., Galavotti, C., O'Reilly, K., Schnell, D., Moore, M., Rugg, D. and Johnson, R. (1991). Evidence for the effect of HIV antibody counselling and testing on risk behaviours. *Journal of the American Medical Association*, Nov. 6, **266**, 17, 2419–29.

Hingson, R., Strunin, L., Carven, D., Mofenson, L., Mangione, T., Berlin, B. et al. (1989). Survey of AIDS knowledge and behaviour changes among Massachusetts adults. *Preventive Medicine*, **18**, 806–16.

Holland, J., Ramazanoglu, C., Scott, S., Sharpe, S. and Thomson, R. (1991). Between embarrassment and trust: young women and the diversity of condom use. In *AIDS Responses Intervention and Care* (P. Aggleton, P. Davies and G. Hart, eds). Basingstoke: Falmer Press.

Holland, J., Ramazanoglu, C., Scott, S., Sharpe, S. and Thomson, R. (1992). Risk, power and the possibility of pleasure: young women and safer sex. *AIDS Care*, **4**, 3, 273–84.

Hooykas, C., van der Linden, M., van Doornam, G., van der Veld, F., van der Pligt, J. et al. (1991). Limited changes in sexual behaviour of heterosexual men and women with multiple partners in the Netherlands. *AIDS Care*, **3**, 21–30.

Ingham, R., Woodcock, A. and Stenner, K. (1991). Getting to know you: young people's knowledge of their partners at first intercourse. *Journal of Community and Applied Social Psychology*, **1**, 117–32.

Janis, I. L. (1967). Effects of fear arousal on attitude change: recent developments in theory and research. In *Advances in Experimental Social Psychology* (L. Berkowitz, ed.) Vol. 3: pp. 166–224. New York: Academic Press.

Johnston, F., Brettle, R., MacCallum, L., Mok, J., Peutherer, J. and Burns, S. (1989). Women's knowledge of their HIV antibody state: its effect on their decision whether to continue the pregnancy. *British Medical Journal*, **300**, 23–4.

Johnson, R., Ostrow, D. and Joseph, J. (1990). Educational strategies for prevention of sexual transmission of HIV. In *Behavioural Aspects of AIDS* (D. Ostrow, ed.). New York: Plenum Press.

Joseph, J., Montgomer, S., Kessler, R., Ostrow, D., Wortmen, C. (1988). Determinants of high risk behaviour and recidivism in gay men. *5th International Conference on AIDS*, Stockholm. Abstract No. 4074.

Keller, M. (1993). Why don't young adults protect themselves against sexual transmission of HIV? Possible answers to a complex question. *AIDS Education and Prevention*, **5**, 3, 220–33.

Kelly, J., Lawrence, J., Hood, H. and Brasfield, T. (1989). Behavioural intervention to reduce AIDS risk activities. *Journal of Consulting and Clinical Psychology*, **57**, 1, 60–7.

Kelly, J., St Lawrence, J. and Brasfield, T. (1991). Predictors of vulnerability to AIDS risk behavior relapse. *Journal of Consultative and Clinical Psychology*, **59**, 163–6.

Kennedy, C., Skurnick, J., Wan, J., Quattrone, G., Sheffet, A. and Quonones, M. (1993). Psychological distress drug and alcohol use as correlates of condom use in HIV serodiscordant heterosexual couples. *AIDS*, **7**, 11, 1493–9.

Kent, V., Davies, M., Deverell, K. and Gottesman, S. (1990). Social interaction routines involved in heterosexual encounters: prelude to first intercourse. Conference paper. *Social Aspects of AIDS*, London.

Kleinot, M. and Rogers, R. (1982). Identifying effective components of alcohol misuse prevention programs. *Journal of Studies in Alcohol*, **43**, 802–11.

Kurth, A. and Hutchinson, M. (1990). Reproductive health policy and HIV: where do women fit in? *Pediatric AIDS and HIV infection: Fetus to Adolescent*, **I**, 121–33.

Leventhal, H. (1970). Findings and theory in the studies of fear communications. In *Advances in Experimental and Social Psychology*, **5**, New York: Academic Press.

Levine, C. and Dubler, N. (1990). HIV and childbearing, 1. Uncertain risks and bitter realities: the reproductive choices of HIV infected women. *The Milbank Quarterly*, **68**, 321–51.

Lupton, D., Chapman, S., Donavon, B. and Mulhall, B. (1992). Attitudes to and use of condoms in multi partnered heterosexuals in Sydney, Australia. *Venereology*, **5**, 2, 41–5.

Manaloto, C., Hayes, C. and Padre, L. L. (1990). Sexual behaviour of Filipino female prostitute after diagnosis of HIV infection. *Southeast Asian Journal of Tropical Medicine and Public Health*, **21**, 2, 301–5.

Mann, J., Nzilambi, N. and Piot, P. (1988). HIV infection and associated risk factors among female prostitutes in Kinshasha, Zaire. *AIDS*, **2**, 249–54.

Martin, D. (1993). Coping with AIDS and AIDS risk reduction efforts among gay men. *AIDS Education and Prevention*, **5**, 2, 104–20.

McCusker, J., Stoddard, A. M. and Mayer, K. H. (1988). Effects of HIV antibody test knowledge on subsequent behaviours in a cohort of homosexually active men. *American Journal of Public Health*, **78**, 462–7.

McCusker, J., Stoddard, A., McDonald, M., Zapka, J. and Mayer, K. (1992). Maintenance of behavioural change in a cohort of homosexually active men. *AIDS*, **6**, 861–8.

McKusick, L., Coates, T., Morin, S., Pollack, L. and Hoff, C. (1990). Longitudinal predictors of reductions in unprotected anal intercourse among gay men in San Francisco: The AIDS Behavioral Research Project. *American Journal of Public Health*, **80**, 978–83.

McKusick, L., Wiley, J. and Coates, T. (1985). Reported changes in the sexual behaviour of men at risk for AIDS. *Public Health Report*, **100**, 622–9.

Miller, D. (1990). Diagnosis and treatment of acute psychological problems related to HIV infection and disease. In *Behavioral Aspects of AIDS*. (D. Ostrow, ed.). New York: Plenum Press.

Ngugi, E., Plummer, F. and Simonsen, J. (1988). Prevention of transmission of Human Immunodeficiency Virus in Africa: Effectiveness of condom promotion and health education among prostitutes. *Lancet*, **2**, 887–90.

Ostrow, D. (1990). *Behavioural Aspects of AIDS*. New York: Plenum Press.

Padian, N., O'Brien, T., Chang, Y., Glass, S. and Francis, D. (1993). Prevention of heterosexual transmission of HIV through couple counselling. *Journal of AIDS*, **6**, 9, 1043–8.

Padian, N., Shiboski, S. and Jewell, N. (1991). Female to male transmission of HIV. *Journal of the American Medical Association*, **266**, 12, 1664–7.

Perkins, D., Leserman, J., Murphy, C. and Evans, D. (1993). Psychosocial predictors of high risk sexual behavior among HIV negative homosexual men. *AIDS Education and Prevention*, **5**, 2, 141–52.

Piot, P., Plummer, F. and Rey, M. (1987). Retrospective seroepidemiology of prostitutes. *Journal of Infectious Diseases*, **155**, 1108–12.

Plummer, F., Moses, S., Jackoniah, O. and Ndinya Achola (1991). Factors affecting female to male transmission of HIV 1. In *AIDS and Women's Reproductive Health* (L. Chen, J. S. Amor and S. Segal, eds). New York: Plenum Press.

Rehmet, S., Staszewski, S., Muller, R., Doerr, H., Bergmann, L., von Wangenheim, G. et al. (1992). Transmission rates and co factors of heterosexual HIV transmission. *7th International Conference on AIDS*, Amsterdam, Abstract No. PoC 4165.

Richardson, D. (1990). AIDS education and women. In *AIDS: Individual, Cultural and Policy Dimensions* (P. Aggleton, P. Davies and H. Hart, eds). Falmer Press.

Ross, M. and Kelaher, M. (1993). Knowledge, attitudes and behaviour. In *AIDS in the Heterosexual Population* (L. Sherr, ed.). Switzerland: Harwood Academic Press.

Selwyn, P., Cater, R. and Schoenbaum, E. (1989). Knowledge of HIV antibody status and decision to continue or terminate pregnancy among intravenous drug users. *Journal of the American Medical Association*, **261**, 3567–71.

Sherr, L. (1987). An evaluation of the UK health education campaign on AIDS. *Psychology and Health*, Nov. 1, 61–72.

Sherr, L. (1990). Fear arousal and AIDS. Do shock tactics work? *AIDS*, **4**, 4, 361–4.

Sherr, L. (1991). *HIV and AIDS in Mothers and Babies*. Oxford: Blackwell Scientific Publications.

Sherr, L. (1993b). HIV testing in pregnancy. In *AIDS and Women* (C. Squire, ed.). London: Sage Publications.

Sherr, L. L. (1994). The psychological impact of fear arousing campaigns. In *Psychology and Promotion of Health*. (J. P. Dauwalder, ed.). Seattle: Hogrefe and Huber.

Sherr, L. and Strong, C. (1991). Safe sex and women. *Genito Urinary Medicine*, **68**, 1.

Sherr, L., Strong, C. and Goldmeier, D. (1990). Sexual behaviour, condom use and prediction in attenders at sexually transmitted disease clinics – implications for counselling. *Counselling Psychology Quarterly*, **3**, 4, 343–52.

Stall, R., Coates, T. and Hoff, C. (1989). Behavioural risk reduction for HIV infection among gay and bisexual men: a review of results from the US. *American Psychology*, **43**, 878–85.

Stratton, P. (1990). Paper presented at FI International Conference on AIDS. San Francisco, Abstract SC 665.

Strunin, L. and Hingson, R. (1993). Adolescents. In *AIDS and the Heterosexual Population* (L. Sherr, ed.). Switzerland: Harwood Academic.

Sunderland, A., Minkoff, H., Handte, J., Moroso, G. and Landesman, S. (1992). The impact of HIV serostatus on reproductive decisions of women. *Obstetrics and Gynaecology*, **79**, 6, 1027–31.

Sutton, S. (1982). Fear arousing communications: a critical examination of theory and research. In *Social Psychology and Behavioral Medicine* (J. Eiser, ed.) pp. 303–37. Chichester: John Wiley.

Sutton, S. (in press). Shock tactics and the myth of the inverted U. Invited editorial, *British Journal of Addiction*.

Sutton, S. and Eiser, J. (1984). The effect of fear arousing communications on cigarette smoking: an expectancy value approach. *Journal of Behavioural Medicine*, **7**, 13–33.

Sutton, S. and Eiser, J. (1990). The decision to wear a seat belt – the role of cognitive factors, fear and prior behaviour. *Psychology and Health*, **4**, 111–23.

Temmerman, M., Mosses, S., Kiragu, D., Fusallah, S., Wamola, I. A. and Piot, P. (1990). Impact of single session post partum counselling on HIV infected women on their subsequent reproductive behaviour. *AIDS Care*, **2**, 3, 247–53.

Treffke, H., Tiggerman, M. and Ross, M. (1992). The relationship between attitude assertiveness and condom use. *Psychology and Health*, **6**, 45–52.

Uitenbroek, D. and McQueen, D. V. (1992). Changing patterns in reported sexual practices in the population: Multiple partners and condom use. *AIDS*, **6**, 587–92.

van de Wijgert, J. and Padian, N. (1993). Heterosexual transmission of HIV. In *AIDS in the Heterosexual Population* (L. Sherr, ed.). Switzerland: Harwood Academic Press.

Walter, H. and Vaughan, R. (1992). AIDS risk reduction among a multiethnic sample of urban high school students. *Journal of the American Medical Association*, **270**, 6, 725–30.

Warner, K. (1981). Cigarette smoking in the 1970s: the impact of the antismoking campaign on consumption. *Science*, **211**, 729–30.

Weinstein, N. D. (1983). Reducing unrealistic optimism about future life events. *Health Psychology*, **2**, 11–20.

Weinstein, N. (1988). The precaution adoption process. *Psychology and Health*, **7**, 355–86.

Wight, D. (1990). Impediments to safer heterosexual sex: a review of research with young people. *AIDS Care*, **4**, 1, 11–24.

Wilkins, H., Alonso, P., Baldeh, S., Cham, M., Corrah, T., Hughes, A. et al. (1989). Knowledge of AIDS: use of condoms and results of counselling subjects with asymptomatic HIV 2 infection in the Gambia. *AIDS Care*, **3**, 1, 247.

Williams, E., Hearst, N. and Udofia, O. (1989). Sexual practices and HIV infection of female prostitutes. 5th International AIDS Conference, Montreal.

Wilson, D. (1993). Preventing transmission of HIV in heterosexual prostitution. In *AIDS in the Heterosexual Population* (L. Sherr, ed.). Switzerland: Harwood Academic.

Wilson, D., Chiroro, P., Lavelle, S. and Mutero, C. (1989). Sex worker: client sex behaviour and condom use in Harare, Zimbabwe. *AIDS Care*, **3**, 1, 269–80.

Wofsy, C. (1988). Women and the acquired immuno deficiency syndrome: An interview. *Women Med*, **149**, 687–90.

Worth, D. (1990). Women at high risk of HIV infection. In *Behavioural Aspects of AIDS* (D. Ostrow, ed.). New York: Plenum Press.

# Female sexuality and reproduction

Jane M. Ussher

Female sexuality has been linked to the capacity to conceive and bear children throughout written history. Women have either been portrayed as uninterested in sex – concerned only to receive sperm passively – or alternatively as having voracious sexual appetites, actively trying to consume as much sperm as possible. Both of these tendencies however are linked to the presumed female desire for pregnancy. In this chapter, Jane Ussher considers female sexuality and our understanding of what is 'normal' sexuality for women. What is 'female sexual dysfunction'? Is vaginal penetration the only sexual act of significance? How can women's sexual needs and experiences be best understood?

## The historical perspective: sexuality and the wandering womb

Sexuality and female reproduction have been irrevocably linked for centuries. Both have been tied to the very essence of what it is to be woman – but rarely to women's advantage. Hippocrates talked of the importance of reproduction in regulating the female constitution – attributing fever, irritability and all manner of other ills to impediments in the 'downward flow of blood' from the womb – menstruation. This lead him to advocate sex – 'cohabitation with a man as quickly as possible' – as cure. Heralding the prescription of pregnancy as a cure for female ailments by a matter of centuries, he also declared that if women 'became pregnant they will be cured'. Plato adopted a similar position, claiming that 'the womb is an animal which longs to bear children'. He apocryphally prophesied that when the womb 'remains barren too long after puberty it becomes distressed and sorely disturbed and straying about the body ... it impedes respiration and brings the sufferer into all manner of anguish and provokes all manner of diseases besides'. Sex and reproduction are again advocated as the cure for disorders afflicting post-pubertal women.

In the witch trials of the fifteenth and sixteenth centuries, reproduction and sexuality were linked in a literally fantastic manner, arguably acting as a justification for misogynistic mass murder. That women were castigated as witches because they were sexual and fertile is evidenced by the declarations of the cleric Reginald Scot in 1584: 'the cause why women are oftener found to be witches than men: they have such an unbridled force of fury and concupiscence naturally that by no means is it possible for them to temper or moderate the same'. The bible of witchcraft, the *Malleus Maleficarum*, is filled with fantasies of the witches' sexual licentiousness – including their having sex with the devil (who was reported to have a three-foot, scaled penis which emitted ice-cold semen), engaging in orgies, and stealing men's penises. Menstruation was at the centre of their crime, of their power and of their fearfulness. For as the worthy cleric Scot continued 'Women are also monthly filled full of superfluous humours, and with them the melancholic blood boils ... to the bewitching of whatsoever it meet'. This has led to the description of the witch trials as 'one million menstrual murders' (Shuttle and Redgrove, 1978).

In the nineteenth century medics who were steeped in the newly evolving discourse of science continued the connection between these peculiarly feminine concerns. Madness, in the form of disorders such as hysteria and neurasthenia, rather than evil, was attributed simultaneously to the womb and to female sexuality. One expert declared that 'in females who become insane the disease is often connected with the peculiarities of their sex' (Haslam, 1917). Another that 'we have to note ... how often sexual feelings arise and display themselves in all forms of insanity' (Maudsley, 1873). The most extreme consequence of this view was the treatment for nervous disorders advocated by Issac Baker Brown – clitoridectomy – literally removing the offending organ as a means of exacting cure (or control). Intercourse, pregnancy and a quiet, obedient marriage were more commonly recommended (Ussher, 1989).

## Female sexuality in the twentieth century

In the twentieth century we might claim to have a more sophisticated and sympathetic understanding of female sexuality, and of its associations with reproduction. We certainly no longer believe that women turn into libidinous witches when they menstruate, or that the womb wanders around the body, inciting illness and discontent. One might argue that the connection between reproduction and sexuality has if anything been severed. That with the exception of the act of conception, reproduction is invariably considered as separate from sex. For example, to speak of connections between menstruation and sex can evoke horror and disgust in many women and men (Ussher, 1989; Laws, 1990). Pregnancy, motherhood and sexuality are equally disconnected, both in theoretical and clinical literature. That pregnancy and lactation may evoke pleasurable sexual feelings is a statement not uncommon in women's self-help literature, but one which appears absent in the mainstream medical and psycho-logical texts, yet these feelings can produce a sensation of discomfort, or fears of sexual abuse, in many women themselves. The splitting of woman into categories of madonna and whore – mother or sexual person – has a widespread and invidious effect. Equally, the notion of the sexual menopausal woman can be seen as a contradiction in terms: sexuality and youth being irrevocably linked.

In research and theory on female sexuality, reproduction is invariably only discussed as a source of dysfunction – where problems associated with menstruation, pregnancy or the menopause are seen to result in sexual diffi-culties. However, as the discussion of female sexuality within the biomedical sciences, including psychology, has for the last hundred years primarily focused on dysfunction, perhaps this is not very surprising.

## Sexuality as dysfunction

Within medicine, psychiatry and psychology, female sexuality is conceptualized as a problem. Analyses of normal or positive female sexuality are strikingly scarce. This may be accounted for by the gender of the researchers, for as one commentator noted 'the issue of female sexuality has been a puzzlement to male social scientists and they have usually elected to ignore it' (Plummer, 1984). Clinicians would appear to be beset by the same puzzlement. For in contrast to the vast body of literature examining the sexuality and sexual problems of men, women are strangely absent from debates of sexual dysfunction. As Cole (1988a) has commented,

> sexual disorders in women, with the possible exception of vaginismus ... are by their very nature less easily categorized because of the more complex nature of women's sexual responses.

Yet the analysis of theoretical and empirical work on sexual dysfunction is essential to any understanding of female sexuality, for by defining a particular phenomenon as dysfunctional, or as sign of illness, we are implicitly stating what we see as the normal boundaries of sexuality. For sexuality is not simply a biological phenomenon – our experience of our sexuality has to be seen in the context of socially constructed definitions of what is normal or abnormal, what is acceptable or unacceptable. These definitions change both across time and across cultures. The biomedical sciences play a central role in defining and maintaining dominant conceptions of female sexuality through their definition and treatment of what is considered a 'sexual problem'.

The three general categories into which female sexual problems are invariably grouped are anorgasmia, inhibited sexual desire/general sexual dysfunction, and vaginismus and dyspareunia. Obtaining accurate information about the epidemiology of these sexual problems is an activity fraught with difficulty, given the inherently private nature of sexuality, and the reluctance of most individuals to discuss their problems with a researcher or clinician. The two avenues of study for those collecting statistics on female sexual problems are studies of clinic attenders, or general surveys of the population. Whilst questions have been raised in relation to the representative nature of the samples of women used, and the validity and reliability of the results presented (Bancroft, 1983) prevalence rates are certainly high.

For example, examining clinic attenders, Masters and Johnson (1966) reported that out of a sample of 342 women 91 per cent experienced orgasmic dysfunction and 9 per cent suffered from vaginismus or dyspareunia. Similarly, Bancroft and Coles (1976) in an analysis of 102 women who attended a sex therapy clinic over a three-year period claimed that 62 per cent of women experienced general sexual problems. Eighteen per cent were anorgasmic and 12 per cent suffered from vaginismus or dyspareunia. Mears (1978) reported that out of 1330 clinic attenders 51 per cent experienced general sexual dysfunction, 22 per cent were anorgasmic and 15 per cent suffered from vaginismus or dyspareunia.

When more general populations of women are questioned, such as through a sexual survey, similarly high rates of problems are suggested. On the subject of anorgasmia in women the estimates range from Hite (1976) who claimed 29 per cent of 3000 women respondents never or almost never achieved orgasm, to Garde and Lunde (1980) who claimed only 4 per cent of their sample of 225 women were anorgasmic. Others report 19 per cent (Chester and Walker, 1980), 15 per cent (Frank, Anderson and Rubinstein, 1978), 7 per cent (Hunt, 1974), 5 per cent (Pietropinto and Sunenauer, 1977), and 4 per cent (Saunders, 1985) were anorgasmic. Vaginismus is reported to affect between 1 and 4 per cent of women (Pasini, 1977; Catalan, Bradley, Gallwey and Hawton, 1981), but exact figures are unknown.

## Diagnosing sexual problems: defining normal sexuality

The statistics on rates of sexual problems should not be accepted unquestioningly – for the very description of certain phenomena as 'dysfunctional' can be placed in doubt. Serious questions can be asked about the definitions of what actually constitutes a 'sexual problem', and conversely, what is 'normal' sexuality. In the nineteenth century, women who showed any signs of a sexual drive – manifested either through masturbation or desire for a man – could be defined as dysfunctional, as the expectation of the time was that a 'good modest' woman was not sexual (Jeffreys, 1987). A woman whose desires were for other women was considered far more of an abberation – her status as deviant beyond dispute. In the late twentieth century such behaviour does not usually come under the diagnostic microscope (although lesbians are still sometimes pathologized for the very existence of their sexual desires; see Kitzinger, 1987). It is women who are *unable* to experience desire or orgasm who are defined as ill. But this categorization today may be as dubious as the categorization of female sexual desire in the nineteenth century as naturally and necessarily absent.

Take the case of anorgasmia – diagnosed if a woman cannot achieve orgasm through intercourse, but not if she cannot achieve orgasm through masturbation; clearly defining orgasm during vaginal penetration as the normal experience for women. A woman's ability (or desire) to give herself autonomous pleasure is not deemed an issue for clinicians, unless she is being taught to masturbate as part of a programme of therapy. However, different surveys suggest that strikingly large numbers of women rarely or never achieve 'unassisted' orgasm during intercourse – up to 80 per cent in one study (Saunders, 1985), suggesting that 'anorgasmia' (as it is narrowly defined) may be experienced by a majority of women, thus challenging the notion of its being deviant or pathological. If Kinsey, Pomeroy, Martin and Gebhard's (1948) estimate that three-quarters of men ejaculate (and therefore terminate intercourse) after only 2 minutes of penetration is in any way accurate, perhaps it is not too surprising that women are anorgasmic without what is euphemistically termed 'assistance'. Is the absence of orgasm during intercourse necessarily a sign of dysfunction? Is it inevitably the woman's problem?

A similar argument could be made about 'inhibited sexual desire', which could imply that a woman who does not desire her partner (or any man) is somehow ill. 'Inhibited sexual desire' describes the problem of a general lack of interest in sex, which is reportedly more common in women than in men (Hawton, 1985; Cole and Dryden, 1988). The manifestations of this disorder include lack of sexual appetite, boredom, anxiety and frequently active avoidance of sex. An often related problem is the condition termed 'impaired sexual arousal' in which women 'fail to become aroused when sexually stimulated by their partners' (Cole and Dryden 1988) even though desire may be present. This again unambiguously refers to a pathology within the woman, rather than looking to her partner, or to the relationship, for reasons for her disinterest or response.

Equally, it could be argued that vaginismus and dyspareunia cannot be unquestioningly considered as simple physical complaints. Vaginismus is manifested by automatic constriction of the muscle of the vagina upon attempt at penetration, resulting in the impossibility of intercourse, or, if the penetration is achieved, extreme pain for the woman. The symptoms of dyspareunia may include vaginal pain, or more general difficulties such as nausea. Both vaginismus and dyspareunia have a clear psychological component, and have often been described as a manifestation of a 'sexual phobia' (e.g. Jehu, 1984). The associated symptoms include anxiety, profuse sweating, nausea, vomiting, diarrhea or palpitations, often precipitated by an act such as a hug or a kiss, as it suggests a progression to sexual intercourse.

Vaginismus is a rare disorder yet it has received more attention from researchers and clinicians than many other sexual difficulties, such as the more common 'disorders of desire'. One explanation for this is that vaginismus provides a more amenable and obvious focus for research and intervention, as it is more easily identified and measured. Within the dominant positivistic framework of psychology and medicine, where measurement and quantification are central to both research, diagnosis, and intervention, and subjective experience is considered to be outside of the realm of 'good science', the more nebulous subjective aspects of female sexuality (such as desire) provide difficulties. Vaginismus may also be deemed more problematic, as it interferes very directly with a man's ability to penetrate the woman whereas absence of desire, or anorgasmia does not. As the main focus of concern of sex therapists and theorists has until relatively recently been heterosexual intercourse (implicitly defining sex *as* intercourse) conditions such as vaginismus and dyspareunia which prevent 'sex' as thus defined are clearly considered more worthy of attention.

Therefore, whilst the literature on sexual dysfunction is informative in that it suggests that sexuality is an arena of difficulty for many women, it also clearly provides an insight into the boundaries of normal sexuality, and the context within which sexuality is socially constructed. The differing explanations put forward to explain sexual difficulties, and the suggestions for treatment, give a further insight into this issue.

## The causes of sexual problems

The major theoretical frameworks adopted to understand both normal and abnormal sexuality are the biological, psychological, and social. Examples of recent research in these areas are included in Tables 11.1 and 11.2. There are a number of implications of these different frameworks. Theorists and therapists inevitably advocate particular courses of treatment on the basis of their own perspective and backgrounds (or in the case of many feminist critics dispute the existence of dysfunction altogether), and so there is no straightforward answer to the question of what is the solution for sexual difficulties. The theories are predominantly unidimensional; looking to biological factors, such as neurotransmitters (i.e. 5HT) (Riley, Riley and Brown, 1986) or testosterone (Dow and Gallagher, 1989), or to social factors, such as sexual abuse (Jehu, 1989) or marital difficulties (Zimmer, 1987) as the root cause of sexual dysfunction. Reproduction has been associated with sexual problems within both psychosocial or biological frameworks (see Table 11.3). For example, it has been argued

**Table 11.1** Biological explanations for sexual problems

| | | |
|---|---|---|
| Alcohol | Pinhas | 1987 |
| | Covington and Kohen | 1984 |
| | Peterson, Hartsock and Lawson | 1984 |
| | Price and Price | 1983 |
| Epilepsy | Ndegwa, Rust, Golombok and Fenwick | 1986 |
| Hyperprolactinaemia | Sobrinho, Sa-Melo, Nunes, Barroco et al. | 1987 |
| Pelvic pain | Black | 1988 |
| Cancer | Bos | 1986 |
| | Weijmar Schultz, Wijma, Van-de-Wiel and Bouma | 1986 |
| | Thomas | 1987 |
| | Andersen and Jochimsen | 1987 |
| Spinal cord lesion | Bregman | 1978 |
| Heart attack | Crenshaw | 1986 |
| | Papadopoulos | 1985 |
| Diabetes | Prather | 1988 |
| | Schreiner-Engel, Schiavi, Vietorisz and Smith | 1987 |
| | Newman and Bertelson | 1986 |
| | Slob, Koster, Radder and Van-der-Werff-ten-Bosch | 1990 |
| | Schreiner-Engel | 1983 |
| Vulvectomy | Stellman | 1984 |
| Urethritis/cystitus | McCormick and Vinson | 1988 |
| | Kaplan and Steege | 1983 |
| Arthritis | Ferguson and Figley | 1979 |

that the menopause is associated with sexual difficulties for women because of the biological consequences of the menopause, which lead to hormonal changes, physical symptoms such as vaginal dryness, hot flushes, and changes in skin tone (see Wilson, 1986). Alternatively, a psychosocial perspective may be adopted, wherein it is the psychological concomitants of the menopause which are seen to be at the root of difficulties – the negative expectations associated with female ageing, the anxiety and depression associated with life stresses, and the sexual difficulties or absence of desire common in long-term relationships which are more common at this time in life (see Chapter 4).

These different aetiological theories clearly have serious implications in terms of the way in which female sexuality is construed, and consequently the way in which problems are treated. For example, take the case of a 50 year old woman presenting to a clinician with 'general sexual dysfunction', manifested by lack of desire. If she is deemed to be suffering from endocrine disorders, or hormonal imbalances associated with the menopause, her treatment may be hormone replacement therapy. If she is deemed to be suffering from problems related to low self-esteem and relationship difficulties, intervention may be psychotherapy or counselling. A social constructionist perspective may result in advice that her 'problem' is understandable and normal, and that she needs to change her view of what is 'sex'.

This is clearly problematic, and will inevitably add to the difficulties of women attempting to gain a wider understanding of their own sexuality and

**Table 11.2** Psychosocial explanations for sexual problems

| Sexual abuse | Charmoli and Athelstan | 1976 |
|---|---|---|
| | Feinauer | 1989 |
| | Jehu | 1989 |
| | Black | 1988 |
| | Kilpatrick | 1986 |
| | Becker, Skinner, Abel and Cichon | 1986 |
| | Resick | 1983 |
| | Gazan | 1986 |
| | Gilbert and Cunningham | 1986 |
| Motivation | Weijmar-Schultz, Wijma, Van-de-Wiel and Bouma | 1986 |
| Personality | Stuart, Hammond and Pett | 1986 |
| Career | Avery-Clark | 1986 |
| Rage | Giovacchini | 1986 |
| No fantasy | Nutter and Condron | 1983 |
| Cognitions | Phinney, Jensen, Olsen and Cundick | 1990 |
| | Alizade | 1988 |
| Contraceptive anxiety | Bruch and Hynes | 1987 |
| Marital problems | Zimmer | 1987 |
| | Stuart, Skinner, Abel and Cichon | 1987 |
| | Whitehead and Mathews | 1986 |
| Men's behaviour | Pietropinto | 1986 |
| | Bancroft | 1984 |
| Psychoanalytic | Richards | 1990 |

problems associated with it. For if different health care professionals give us completely different explanations and treatments for distress, how are we to decide whose advice to follow? It might be argued that to posit a unidimensional explanation for sexual problems – to adopt *either* a solely psychosocial or biological framework – is naïve. For whilst in a minority of cases there may be a clear aetiological root for a woman's sexual difficulties, it is unlikely that one psychosocial or biological factor is the sole cause of difficulty. For example, within a biological view, it is argued that sexual problems are related to some physical illness or to endocrine function, as is illustrated above (see Table 11.1). Cancer, diabetes, or the menopause may seem simple causes of sexual difficulties – a consistent correlation between identified clinical populations and rates of sexual problems allowing for a strong case to be made for generalizable theories. Yet it is not so simple. It is not enough to posit a physical (or psychological) cause for a sexual difficulty and then treat it out of context of any other facet of a woman's experience. For example, cancer itself does not *cause* sexual difficulties, but the concomitant physical, psychological and social factors associated with disease may result in symptomatology.

The same critique could be levelled at models which might seem diametrically opposite, such as a psychosocial model which posits that sexual abuse is the main precursor of sexual difficulty. Sexual abuse may clearly lead to later sexual difficulties in women, as attested by analyses of both clinical and more general population samples (see Table 11.2). But it is not enough to posit that

**Table 11.3** Reproduction and sexual problems

| Hormones | Schreiner-Engel | 1989 |
|---|---|---|
|  | Benton and Wastell | 1986 |
|  | Whitehead and Mathews | 1986 |
|  | Melman | 1983 |
| Menstruation | Morris, Udry, Khan-Dawood and Dawood | 1987 |
|  | Bancroft, Sanders, Davidson and Warner | 1983 |
| Menopause | Cutler, Garcia and McCoy | 1987 |
|  | Myers and Morokoff | 1986 |
|  | Channon and Ballinger | 1986 |
|  | Sherwin, Gelfand and Brender | 1985 |
|  | Leiter | 1983 |
| Osteoporosis | Reyniak | 1987 |
| Hysterectomy | Ananth | 1983 |
| Post-partum | Debrovner and Shubin | 1985 |
| Pregnancy | Elliott and Watson | 1985 |
|  | Alder and Bancroft | 1983 |

sexual abuse in childhood inevitably leads to anxiety around sexuality in adult women – this consequence is affected by a myriad of factors including the silence associated with sexuality, the differential power relations between men and women, the positioning of the individual woman within a heterosexual culture, and the many other psychological and physical consequences of sexual abuse. Women who have been abused have been shown to be at risk of depression, anxiety, self-injurious behaviour or attempts to commit suicide (Browne and Finkelhor, 1986). They often experience a distorted sense of reality as the victimization creates a negative sense of the world, where little seems meaningful and where the woman herself feels weak, needy, frightened and out of control. The woman's whole image of the world, and of herself, can become imbued with negative overtones. It is this complex interaction which affects her sexual identity and her sexual response.

In an attempt to move away from the one dimensional view, a number of psychologists have advocated a more integrated or multidimensional approach,

**Table 11.4** Multi-modal therapies for sexual problems

| Dow and Gallagher, 1989 | Testosterone vs counselling (latter more effective). 30 couples; sexual unresponsiveness in female partner |
|---|---|
| Golubtsova and Polishchuk, 1988 | Multi-modal drugs/therapy/acupuncture/diet. 90 women with progressive schizophrenia |
| Whitehead and Mathews, 1986 | M & J counselling plus placebo or testosterone effective. 48 couples, lack of female sexual response |
| Riley, Riley and Brown, 1986 | Review of hormonal/chemical control of sexual desire in women |

**Table 11.5** Psychosocial therapies for sexual dysfunction

| | |
|---|---|
| Milan, Kilmann and Bowland, 1988 | Group therapy: 38 women, orgasmic dysfunction |
| Gazan, 1986 | Package: relaxation training, cognitive restructuring, treatment of the sexual dysfunctions. 5 sexually abused women and their partners, who sought therapy |
| Zimmer, 1987 | Cognitive-behavioural therapy: marital therapy vs relaxation/ information (marital more effective). 28 couples, wives' secondary sexual dysfunction |
| Whitehead, Mathews and Ramage, 1987 | Cojoint M & J therapy vs women-focused method (both effective). 44 couples, lack of sexual response in women |
| Jonsson and Byers, 1986 | Graduated modelling in sexually anxious woman. One 22 year old woman |
| Becker, Skinner, Abel and Cichon, 1984 | Time limited, behaviourally oriented treatment package, 68 sexually abused women |
| Adkins and Jehu, 1985 | Behavioural treatment, 6 couples, woman anorgasmic |
| Nairne and Hemsley, 1983 | Directed masturbatory training. Review |
| Rust and Golombok, 1990 | Stress reduction and global approach for women. Review |

generally taking the position espoused by Bancroft (1983) that sexuality must be conceived of within a psychosomatic circle, where physiology and cognitions interact, implying that treatment should operate on a number of different levels. This approach acknowledges the influence of both biological and social factors, ideally not privileging one above the other. The adoption of a biopsychosocial framework has also led to a move away from unidimensional treatments, as is evidenced by the number of recent research studies examining the impact of multi-factorial treatment packages (Table 11.4). At the same time, the recognition that many women presenting with sexual difficulties are not suffering from any physical problem has led to the development of psychological treatment packages (Table 11.5).

## Contextualizing female sexuality

The discussion thus far has concentrated primarily on sexual problems. This is not coincidental. For whilst outside of psychology scholars have deconstructed the discourse associated with sexuality (Foucault, 1979) or provided critical analyses of the relationship, the social construction of sexuality and the control of women (Jeffreys, 1990; Nicolson, 1993), those working within the biomedical disciplines of psychology and medicine appear to have reduced sexuality to its component parts. To 'incidence and frequency', to the cataloguing of dysfunctional symptoms, or to a variable able to be manipulated and measured in exact experimentation in research which is then used as supporting evidence for psychological theories and therapies. Yet we must beg the question, as this research is so esoteric or abstract, viewing female sexuality out of any social context, can it be accepted unquestioningly?

This is never more clear than in the laboratory based experimental research wherein sexuality is reduced to the level of 'vaginal pulse amplitude' (e.g. Rogers et al., 1985) or where women's erotic sensitivity is measured by 'means of the systematic digital stimulation of the vaginal walls' (Alzate and Londono, 1984). Experimental research on female sexuality (see Ussher, 1993) reduces sexuality to the status of abstract experimental variables, the woman herself invisible behind the attention given to carefully selected aspects of her sexuality which are dissected and discussed. The vibration of her vaginal walls is of interest, her subjective experience of her sexuality ignored. Whether these intrusive experiments are meaningful or justifiable may be questionable, but the fact that this genre of research forms the bulk of psychological research on female sexuality is evidence of the denial of subjectivity at the expense of exact experimentation in mainstream psychology.

This approach is not confined to the experimental psychologists, for throughout the academic and clinical literature on the subject of sexual problems in women there is a curious distance and use of language which is devoid of any notion of the woman's own experience. It is always clinical, cool and objective. Take this recent description of dyspareunia and vaginismus:

> dyspareunia in the female (pain in the vagina during intercourse) and vaginismus can be viewed as similar problems with varying degrees of intensity. They range from a dyspareunia of mild discomfort, through serious and perhaps intolerable pain, to vaginismus where the reflex contracture of the peri-vaginal muscles effectively prevents penetration by the penis. In more serious cases, any attempt to touch or approach the vagina leads to powerful reflex adduction of the thighs, thus precluding even the possibility of attempted penetration.

This analysis focuses on physical reactions and complaints to the exclusion of any analysis of the psychological or social factors associated with the woman's distress. That penetration *could* be attempted in such a situation is astounding. The underlying assumptions about male and female sexual relationships in such a scenario are not even hinted at in the clinical analysis; female sexuality is again positioned as something to be assessed, manipulated and treated, with successful accomplishment of intercourse the end goal – at all costs.

It is this focus on sex as intercourse, and on the categorization of discrete aspects of sexuality as functional or dysfunctional, reinforcing the taxonomic systems of the psychologists and medics, which has come under greatest criticism from a number of disciplines. It has been argued that sexuality is an important arena of social control, and that since the nineteenth century the adoption of medical and psychological models as a means of categorizing sexual behaviour have acted as 'a means of access both to the life of the body and the life of the species' (Foucault, 1979). This process of control of women through sexuality has clearly been present for centuries, as was demonstrated at the beginning of the chapter in the edicts of Plato, Hippocrates and the experts on witchcraft. But it was in the nineteenth century through the 'hysterisization of sex' (Foucault, 1979) that female sexuality was defined as inherently dysfunctional.

More recently, feminist critics have taken up this analysis (see Nicolson, 1993), seeing that psychological theory on female sexuality functions to maintain women's sexual subordination. As Sheila Jeffreys (1990) has argued,

The setting up of the marriage guidance council, the work of sexologists and the development of sex therapy are all instances of how men's power over women was to be supported through the regulation of marital sex.

Theories of sexuality and definitions of sexual dysfunction within psychology have been seen as being based on misogynistic theorizing, functioning to pathologize women who do not seek or achieve pleasure within the phallocentrically biased heterosexual relationship. Sex therapy has been positioned as objectifying for women, 'tinkering with the husband/wife relationship so as to bolster the man's power and subordinate the woman' (Jeffreys, 1990). It is argued that some women's understandable physical reaction to heterosexual sex, repugnance, is pathologized through being labelled as vaginismus, a syndrome elevated to the status of phobia, as a 'dread of the penis' (Jeffreys, 1990). And that it is only when the woman cannot perform (i.e. receive the penis) during intercourse that her sexual difficulties are taken seriously. Underlying theories and therapies is 'the assumption of the primacy of erections over other sexual concerns' (Stock, 1988). And whilst the 'inability of the male to have a cylindrical tube of flesh between the legs become sufficiently rigid to insert in a vagina' (Stock, 1988) is a major sexual dysfunction, problems with emotional intimacy, communication about sex, or female dissatisfaction with intercourse as the focus of sexual activity are invariably ignored. So whilst psychologists who theorize about female sexuality are maligned for narrowly defining what is legitimately a 'problem' for women (i.e. intercourse not intimacy), the therapists are condemned for being merely 'dedicated to the maintenance of marriage and heterosexuality' (Jackson, 1984).

This narrow definition of sexuality and sexual dysfunction marginalizes the needs of many women. For example, lesbian women, women with a disability, or older women can all be said to be absent from the agenda of the sex experts. To a degree, this is changing. There is increasing awareness that sexuality cannot be considered within the narrow boundaries of heterosexual relationships between two people of reproductive age. It is being recognized that attention needs to be given to the sexual needs and concerns of younger women, lesbians, women with children, older women, and women with a disability (Ussher and Baker, 1993; Choi and Nicolson, 1994) amongst others. There is also increasing attention given to women's subjective experience of sexuality and of sexual problems (Hollway, 1989), and consequently a move away from experimental research on sex, or narrow models of therapy that focus on vaginal penetration. The critical arguments raging outside of the biomedical sciences for decades appear to be being heard inside the disciplines of psychology and medicine. Theory and therapy is broadening to encompass an acknowledgement of the social construction of sexuality, and the complex psychological, social and physical roots of both sexual difficulties and sexual satisfaction. It is with this broad framework that understanding of the relationship between reproduction and sexuality will continue to develop.

## Applications

### 1. Defining sex and sexuality
There is more to sex than the penetration of a vagina by a penis. Research and therapy which approaches sex in this mechanistic way distorts definitions of sexual dysfunction and marginalizes the needs and experiences of many women. A broader definition of sex and sexuality is required if these needs are to be met.

### 2. Multidimensional approaches to intervention
Sexuality is influenced by biological, psychological and social factors, which are equally important. Approaches to therapy need to consider not only the physiological aspects of any perceived dysfunction but also the social context of the relationship in which it occurs and the cognitions associated with it.

## Further reading

Bancroft, J. (1989). *Human Sexuality and its Problems*. (2nd edn). Edinburgh: Churchill Livingstone.
Choi, P. and Nicolson, P. (eds) (1994). *Female Sexuality*. Hemel Hempstead: Harvester Wheatsheaf.
Ussher, J. and Baker, C. (eds) (1993). *Psychological Perspectives on Sexual Problems: New Directions for Theory and Practice*. London: Routledge.

## References

Adkins, E. and Jehu, D. (1985). Analysis of a treatment program for primary orgastic dysfunction. *Behaviour Research and Therapy*, **23**, 2, 119–26.
Alder, E. and Bancroft, J. (1983). Sexual behaviour of lactating women: A preliminary communication. *Journal of Reproductive and Infant Psychology*, **1**, 2, 47–52.
Alexander and Selesnick (1966). *The History of Psychiatry*. London: Allen and Unwin.
Alizade, A. M. (1988). Ensayo psicoanalitico sobre el orgasmo femenino. (A psychoanalytic essay on the subject of female orgasm.) *Revista de Psicoanalisis*, **45**, 2, 337–52.
Alzate, H. and Londono, M. L. (1984). Vaginal erotic sensitivity. *Journal of Sex and Marital Therapy*, **10**, 1, 49–56.
Ananth, J. (1983). Hysterectomy and sexual counselling. *Psychiatric Journal of the University of Ottawa*, **8**, 4, 213–7.
Andersen, B. L. and Jochimsen, P. R. (1987). 'Research design and strategy for studying psychological adjustment to cancer': Reply to Thomas. *Journal of Consulting and Clinical Psychology*, **55**, 1, 122–4.
Avery-Clark, C. (1986). Sexual dysfunction and disorder patterns of husbands of working and nonworking women. *Journal of Sex and Marital Therapy*, **12**, 4, 282–96.
Bancroft, J. (1974). *Deviant Sexual Behaviour: Modification and Assessment*. Oxford: Clardendon Press.
Bancroft, J. (1983). *Human Sexuality and its Problems*. London: Churchill Livingstone.

Bancroft, J. (1984). Interaction of psychosocial and biological factors in marital sexuality: Differences between men and women. *British Journal of Guidance and Counselling*, **12**, 1, 62–71.

Bancroft, J. and Coles, L. (1976). Three years' experience in a sexual problems clinic. *British Medical Journal*, **1**, 1575–7.

Bancroft, J., Sanders, D., Davidson, D. and Warner, P. (1983). Mood, sexuality, hormones and the menstrual cycle: III. Sexuality and the role of androgens. *Psychosomatic Medicine*, **45**, 6, 509–16.

Becker, J. V., Skinner, L. J., Abel, G. G. and Cichon, J. (1984). Time limited therapy with sexually dyfunctional sexually assaulted women. *Journal of Social Work and Human Sexuality*, **3**, 1, 97–115.

Becker, J. V., Skinner, L. J., Abel, G. G. and Cichon, J. (1986). Level of postassault sexual functioning in rape and incest victims. *Archives of Sexual Behavior*, **15**, 1, 37–49.

Benton, D. and Wastell, V. (1986). Effects of androstenol on human sexual arousal. *Biological Psychology*, **22**, 2, 141–7.

Black, J. S. (1988). Sexual dysfunction and dyspareunia in the otherwise normal pelvis. *Sexual and Marital Therapy*, **3**, 2, 213–21.

Bos, G. (1986). Sexuality of gynaecological cancer patients: Quantity and quality. *Journal of Psychosomatic Obstetrics and Gynaecology*, **5**, 3, 217–24.

Bregman, S. (1978). Sexual adjustment of spinal cord injured women. *Sexuality and Disability*, **1**, 85–92.

Browne, A. and Finkelhor, D. (1986). Impact of child sexual abuse: a review of the literature. *Psychological Bulletin*, **99**, 1, 66–77.

Bruch, M. A., Hynes, M. J. (1987). Heterosocial anxiety and contraceptive behavior. *Journal of Research in Personality*, **21**, 3, 343–60.

Catalan, J., Bradley, M., Gallwey, J. and Hawton, K. (1981). Sexual dysfunction and psychiatric morbidity in patients attending a clinic for sexually transmitted diseases. *British Journal of Psychiatry*, **138**, 292–6.

Channon, L. D. and Ballinger, S. E. (1986). Some aspects of sexuality and vaginal symptoms during menopause and their relations to anxiety and depression. *British Journal of Medical Psychology*, **59**, 2, 173–80.

Charmoli, M. C., Athelstan, G. T. (1988). Incest as related to sexual problems in women. *Journal of Psychology and Human Sexuality*, **1**, 1, 53–66.

Chester, R. and Walker, C. (1980). Sexual experience and attitudes of British women. In *Changing Patterns of Sexual Behaviour* (W. H. G. Armytage, R. Chester, and J. Peel, eds). London: Academic Press.

Choi, P. and Nicolson, P. (1994). Female sexuality. Hemel Hempstead: Harvester Wheatsheaf.

Cole, M. (1988a). Normal and dysfunctional sexual behaviour: frequencies and incidences. In *Sex Therapy in Britain* (M. Cole and W. Dryden, eds). Milton Keynes: Open University Press.

Cole, M. (1988b). Sex therapy for individuals. In *Sex Therapy in Britain* (M. Cole and W. Dryden, eds). Milton Keynes: Open University Press.

Cole, M. and Dryden, W. (1988). Sexual dysfunction: an introduction. In *Sex Therapy in Britain* (M. Cole and W. Dryden, eds). Milton Keynes: Open University Press.

Cooper, G. F. (1988). The psychological methods of sex therapy. In *Sex Therapy in Britain* (M. Cole and W. Dryden, eds). Milton Keynes: Open University Press.

Covington, S. S. and Kohen, J. (1984). Women, alcohol, and sexuality, *Advances in Alcohol and Substance Abuse*, **4**, 1, 41–56.

Crenshaw, T. L. (1986). A woman's persistent fear of sex two years after a heart attack. *Medical Aspects of Human Sexuality*, **20**, 12, 50–51.

Cutler, W. B., Garcia, C. R. and McCoy, N. (1987). Perimenopausal sexuality. *Archives of Sexual Behavior*, **16**, 3, 225–34.

Debrovner, C. H. and Shubin, R. (1985). Pregnancy and postpartum: II. Postpartum sexual concerns. *Medical Aspects of Human Sexuality*, **19**, 5, 84–90.

Dow, M. G. and Gallagher, J. (1989). A controlled study of combined hormonal and psychological treatment for sexual unresponsiveness in women. *British Journal of Clinical Psychology*, Sept, **28**, 3, 201–12.

Elliott, S. A. and Watson, J. P. (1985). Sex during pregnancy and the first postnatal year. *Journal of Psychosomatic Research*, **29**, 5, 541–8.

Feinauer, L. L. (1989). Sexual dysfunction in women sexually abused as children. *Contemporary Family Therapy: An International Journal*, **11**, 4, 299–309.

Ferguson, K. and Figley, B. (1979). Sexuality and rheumatic disease: a study. *Sexuality and Disability*, **2**, 130–8.

Foucault, M. (1979). *The History of Sexuality*, Vol. 1. London: Allen Lane.

Frank, E., Anderson, C. and Rubinstein, D. (1978). Frequency of sexual dysfunction in 'normal' couples. *New England Journal of Medicine*, **299**, 111–15.

Garde, K. and Lunde, I. (1980). Female sexual behaviour: a study in a random sample of 40 year old women. *Maturitas*, **2**, 225–40.

Gazan, M. (1986). An evaluation of a treatment package designed for women with a history of sexual victimization in childhood and sexual dysfunctions in adulthood. Special Issue: Women and mental health. *Canadian Journal of Community Mental Health*, **5**, 2, 85–102.

Gilbert, B. and Cunningham, J. (1986). Women's postrape sexual functioning: Review and implications for counselling. *Journal of Counselling and Development*, **65**, 2, 71–3.

Giovacchini, P. L. (1986). Promiscuity in adolescents and young adults. *Medical Aspects of Human Sexuality*, **20**, 5, 24–31.

Golubtsova, L. I. and Polishchuk, Y. I. (1988). Multiple modality therapy of sexual disorders in women with slowly progressive schizophrenia. *Zhurnal Nevropatologii i Psikhiatrii*, **88**, 2, 110–14.

Haslam, J. (1917). *Considerations on the Moral Management of the Insane*. London: R. Hunter.

Hawton, K. (1985). *Sex Therapy: A Practical Guide*. Oxford: Oxford University Press.

Hite, S. (1976). *The Hite Report*. New York: Macmillan.

Hollway, W. (1989). *Subjectivity and Method in Psychology*. London: Sage.

Hunt, M. (1974). *Sexual Behaviour in the 1970s*. Chicago: Playboy Press.

Jackson, M. (1984). Sex research and the construction of sexuality: a tool for male supremacy? *Women's Studies International Forum*, **7**, 43–51.

Jeffreys, S. (1987). *The Sexuality Debates*. London: Routledge.

Jeffreys, S. (1990). *Anticlimax: A Feminist Perspective on the Sexual Revolution*. London: The Women's Press.

Jehu, D. (1984). Impairment of sexual behaviour in non-human primates. In *The Psychology of Sexual Diversity* (K. Howells, ed.). Oxford: Basil Blackwell.

Jehu, D. (1989). Sexual dysfunctions among women clients who were sexually abused in childhood. *Behavioural Psychotherapy*, **17**, 1, 53–70.

Jonsson, B. D. and Byers, E. S. (1986). Treatment of sexual anxiety with graduate modelling. *Journal of Sex Education and Therapy*, **12**, 1, 60–4.

Kaplan, D. L., Steege, J. F. (1983). The urethral syndrome: Sexual components. *Sexuality and Disability*, **6**, 2, 78–82.

Kilpatrick, A. C. (1986). Some correlates of women's childhood sexual experiences: A retrospective study. *Journal of Sex Research*, **22**, 2, 221–42.

Kinsey, A. C., Pomeroy, W. B., Martin, C. E. and Gebhard, P. H. (1948). *Sexual Behaviour in the Human Male*. Philadelphia and London: W. B. Saunders Co.

Kitzinger, C. (1987). *The Social Construction of Lesbianism*. London: Sage.

Klassen, A. D. and Wilsnack, S. C. (1986). Sexual experience and drinking among women in a U.S. national survey. *Archives of Sexual Behavior* **15**, 5, 363–92.

Laws, S. (1990). *Issues of Blood*. London: Chapman and Hall.

Leiter, E. (1983). Urethritis: Clinical manifestations and inter-relationship with intercourse and therapy. *Sexuality and Disability*, **6**, 2, 72–7.

Masters, W. H. and Johnson, V. E. (1966). *Human Sexual Response*. Boston, MA: Little, Brown and Co.

Maudsley, H. (1873). *Body and Mind*. London: Macmillian.

McCormick, N. B. and Vinson, R. K. (1988). Sexual difficulties experienced by women with interstitial cystitis. (Special issue: Women and sex therapy). *Women and Therapy*, **7**, 2–3, 109–19.

Mears, E. (1978). Sexual problem clinics: an assessment of the work of 26 doctors trained by the Institute of Psychosexual Medicine. *Public Health*, **92**, 218–33.

Melman, A. (1983). The interaction of urinary tract infection and sexual intercourse in women. *Sexuality and Disability*, **6**, 2, 93–8.

Milan, R. J., Kilmann, P. R. and Boland, J. P. (1988). Treatment outcome of secondary orgasmic dysfunction: A two- to six-year follow up. *Archives of Sexual Behavior* **17**, 6, 463–80.

Mitchell, J. (1974). *Psychoanalysis and Feminism*. London: Allen Lane.

Morris, N. M., Udry, J. R., Khan-Dawood, F. and Dawood, M. Y. (1987). Marital sex frequency and midcycle female testosterone. *Archives of Sexual Behavior*, **16**, 1, 27–37.

Myers, L. S. and Morokoff, P. J. (1986). Physiological and subjective sexual arousal in pre and postmenopausal women and postmenopausal women taking replacement therapy. *Psychophysiology*, **23**, 3, 283–92.

Nairne, K. D. and Hemsley, D. R. (1983). The use of directed masturbation training in the treatment of primary anorgasmia. *British Journal of Clinical Psychology*, **22**, 4, 2833–94.

Ndegwa, D., Rust, J., Golombok, S. and Fenwick, P. (1986). Sexual problems in epileptic women. *Sexual and Marital Therapy* **1**, 2, 175–7.

Newman, A. S. and Bertelson, A. D. (1986). Sexual dysfunction in diabetic women. *Journal of Behavioural Medicine*, **9**, 3, 261–70.

Nicolson, P. (1993). Public values and private beliefs: Why do women refer themselves for sex therapy? In *Psychological perspectives on Sexual Problems: New Directions for Theory and Practice* (J. M. Ussher and C. Baker, eds). London: Routledge.

Nutter, D. E. and Condron, M. K. (1983). Sexual fantasy and activity patterns of females with inhibited sexual desire versus normal controls. *Journal of Sex and Marital Therapy*, **9**, 4, 276–82.

Papadopoulos, C. (1985). Sexuality of women after myocardial infarction. *Medical Aspects of Human Sexuality*, **19**, 3, 215–23.

Pasini, W. (1977). Unconsummated and partially consummated marriage as sources of procreative failure. In *Handbook of Sexology* (J. Money and H. Musaph, eds). Amsterdam: Elsevier.

Peterson, J. S., Hartsock, N., Lawson, G. (1984). Sexual dissatisfaction of female alcoholics. *Psychological Reports*, **55**, 3, 744–46.

Phinney, V. G., Jensen, L. C., Olsen, J. A., Cundick, B. (1990). The relationship between early development and psychosexual behaviours in adolescent females. *Adolescence*, **25**, 98, 321–32.

Pietropinto, A. (1986). Male contributions to female sexual dysfunction. *Medical Aspects of Human Sexuality*, **20**, 12, 84–91.

Pietropinto, A. and Simenauer, J. (1977). *Beyond the Male Myth. A Nationwide Survey*. New York: Times Books.

Pinhas, V. (1987). Sexual dysfunction in women alcoholics. *Medical Aspects of Human Sexuality*, **21**, 6, 97–101.

Plummer, K. (1984). Sexual diversity: a sociological perspective. In *The Psychology of Sexual Diversity* (K. Howells, ed.). Oxford: Basil Blackwell.

Prather, R. C. (1988). Sexual dysfunction in the diabetes female: A review. *Archives of Sexual Behavior*, **17**, 3, 277–84.

Price, J. A. and Price, J. H. (1983). Alcohol and sexual functioning: A review. *Advances in Alcohol and Substance Abuse*, **2**, 4, 43–56.

Resick, P. A. (1983). The rape reaction: Research findings and implications for intervention. *Behavior Therapist*, **6**, 7, 129–32.

Reyniak, J. V. (1987). Sexual and other concerns of the woman with osteoporosis. *Medical Aspects of Human Sexuality*, **21**, 1, 161–7.

Richards, A. (1990). Female fetishes and female perversions. *Psychoanalytic Review*, **77**, 1, 11–23.

Riley, A. J. and Riley, E. J. (1986). The effect of single dose diazepam on female sexual response induced by masturbation. *Sexual and Marital Therapy*, **1**, 1, 49–53.

Riley, A. J., Riley, E. J. and Brown, P. T. (1986). Biological aspects of sexual desire in women. *Sexual and Marital Therapy*, **1**, 1, 35–42.

Rogers, G. S., Van-de-Castle, R. L., Evans, W. S. et al. (1985) Vaginal pulse amplitude response patterns during erotic conditions and sleep. *Archives of Sexual Behaviour*, **14**, 4, 377–42.

Rust, J. and Golombok, S. (1990). Stress and marital discord: Some sex differences. *Stress Medicine*, **6**, 1, 25–7.

Saunders, D. (1985). *The Woman's Book of Love and Sex*. London: Sphere.

Schreiner-Engel, P. (1983). Diabetes mellitus and female sexuality. *Sexuality and Disability*, **6**, 2, 83–92.

Schreiner-Engel, P., Schiavi, R. C., Vietorisz, D. and Smith, H. (1987). The differential impact of diabetes type on female sexuality. *Journal of Psychosomatic Research*, **31**, 1, 23–33.

Schreiner-Engel, P., Schiavi, R. C., White, D. and Ghizzani, A. (1989). Low sexual desire in women: The role of reproductive hormones. *Hormones and Behavior*, **23**, 2, 221–34.

Sherwin, B. B., Gelfand, M. M. and Brender, W. (1985). Androgen enhances sexual motivation in females: A prospective, crossover study of sex steroid administration in the surgical menopause. *Psychosomatic Medicine*, **47**, 4, 339–51.

Shuttle, P. and Redgrove, P. (1978). *The Wise Wound: Menstruation and Every Woman*. London: Gollanz.

Slob, A. K., Koster, J., Radder, J. K. and Van-der-Werff-ten-Bosch, J. J. (1990). Sexuality and psychophysiological functioning in women with diabetes mellitus. *Journal of Sex and Marital Therapy*, **16**, 2, 59–69.

Sobrinho, L. G., Sa-Melo, P., Nunes, M. C., Barroco, L. E. (1987). Sexual dysfunction in hyper-prolactinaemic women: Effect of bromocriptine. *Journal of Psychosomatic Obstetrics and Gynaecology*, **6**, 1, 43–8.

Stellman, R. E. (1984). Psychological effects of vulvectomy. *Psychosomatics*, **25**, 10, 779–83.

Stock, W. (1988). Propping up phallocracy: a feminist critique of sex therapy and research. *Women and Therapy*, **2–3**, 23–41.

Stuart, F. M., Hammond, D. C. and Pett, M. A. (1986). Psychological characteristics of women with inhibited sexual desire. *Journal of Sex and Marital Therapy*, **12**, 2, 108–15.

Stuart, F. M., Hammond, D. C. and Pett, M. A. (1987). Inhibited sexual desire in women. *Archives of Sexual Behavior*, **16**, 2, 91–106.

Stuntz, R. C. (1986). Physical obstructions to coitus in women. *Medical Aspects of Human Sexuality*, **20**, 2, 117–34.

Taylor, S. E. (1983). Adjustment to threatening events: A theory of cognitive adaptation. *American Psychologist*, **38**, 1161–73.

Thomas, J. (1987). Problems in a study of the sexual response of women with cancer: Comment on Andersen and Jochimsen. *Journal of Consulting and Clinical Psychology*, **55**, 1, 120–21.

Ussher, J. M. (1989). *The Psychology of the Female Body*. London: Routledge.

Ussher, J. M. (1991). *Women's Madness: Misogyny or Mental Illness*. Hemel Hempstead: Harvester Wheatsheaf.

Ussher, J. M. (1990). The future of sex and marital therapy in the face of widespread criticism: caught between the devil and the deep blue sea. *Counselling Psychology Quarterly*, **3**, 4, 317–24.

Ussher, J. M. (1993). The construction of female sexual problems: regulating sex, regulating women. In *Psychological Perspectives on Sexual Problems: New Directions for Theory and Practice* (J. M. Ussher and C. Baker, eds). London: Routledge.

Ussher, J. and Baker, C. (eds) (1993). *Psychological Perspectives on Sexual Problems: New Directions for Theory and Practice*. London: Routledge.

Weeks, J. (1990). *Sex, Politics and Society: The Regulation of Sexuality since 1800*. London: Longmans.

Weijmar-Schultz, W. C., Wijma, K., Van-de-Wiel, H. B., Bouma, J. (1986). Sexual rehabilitation of radical vulvectomy patients: A pilot study. *Journal of Psychosomatic Obstetrics and Gynaecology*, **5**, 2, 119–26.

Whitehead, A. and Mathews, A. (1986). Factors related to successful outcome in the treatment of sexually unresponsive women. *Psychological Medicine*, **16**, 2, 373–8.

Whitehead, A., Mathews, A. and Ramage, M. (1987). The treatment of sexually unresponsive women. A comparative evaluation. *Behaviour Research and Therapy*, **25**, 3, 195–205.

Wilson, G. D. (1988). The sociobiological basis of sexual dysfunction. In *Sex Therapy in Britain* (M. Cole and W. Dryden, eds). Milton Keynes: Open University Press.

Wilson, R. A. (1966). *Feminine Forever*. New York: M. Evans.

Wilson, R. J., Beecham, C. T. and Carrington, E. R. (1975). *Obstetrics and Gynaecology*, St. Louis: Mosby.

Zimmer, D. (1987). Does marital therapy enhance the effectiveness of treatment for sexual dysfunction? *Journal of Sex and Marital Therapy*, **13**, 3, 193–209.

# Index

Gender
  adolescence and, 24–5
  behaviourism and social learning, 6–7
  biological determinism, 4–5
  cognitive developmental approach, 7–8
  compared to sex, 22
  constancy, 7
  contemporary interest, 1
  contraceptive use, 127, 128, 132
  essentialist perspectives, 3–6
  identity, 7
  Kohlberg *et al.* on, 7–8
  lenses of, 10
  post-modern approaches, 11–12
  reproductive decisions, 112
  role, 23
  social constructionism, 10–11
  stability, 7
  typing, 7, 9
Gender schema theory, 9–10
Growth spurt, 17
Gynaecological procedures
  definition, 78
  future research, 87–8
  psychological implications, 78, 87
  psychological preparation, 85, 86 table
    efficacy, 85–6
    summary, 87
  psychosocial effects, 81–2
  *see also* specific procedures

Haringey
  abortion in, 108
  family planning services, 110–11
  fertility rate, 108
  number of births, 108
  population characteristics, 108
Health belief model, premarital contraception,
    125
Hindus, 112
Hippocrates, 167
HIV/AIDS
  pregnancy, 156
  prevention, early effectors, 154
  sexual behaviour, 155
    attitudes and changes in, 160–1
    in context of relationship, 159
    counselling and, 161–2
    early attempts to affect, 154
    fear arousal in education campaigns,
      158–9, 162
    health belief models, 159–60
    intervention studies, 158–9
    knowledge, attitude and behaviour studies,
      157–8
    precaution adoption model, 159
    psychological approaches, 156–61
    research into, 155
    self-perception of vulnerability, 160, 161
    social learning theory, 160

  social skills, 161, 162
  theoretical contributions, 159–60
  theory of reasoned action, 160
  in women, 155–6
Hormone replacement therapy (HRT), 60, 61,
    *see also* Oestrogen therapy
Hot flushes, 60, 65–6, 72
HRT, *see* Hormone replacement therapy
Human immunodeficiency virus (HIV)
  adolescence, effect on, 26
  description, 154
  effects of diagnosis, 154
  prevention, early messages, 154
  sexual behaviour, research, 155
  transmission, male to female/female to male,
    155
  *see also* HIV/AIDS
Hysterectomy, 80
  pyschological effects, 84
  sexuality, 84
  total abdominal, 77
  as unnecessary surgery, 84–5
Hysterosalpingography, 79
Hysteroscopy, 79
  with D &, C, 80

Identity
  coherent, 29
  diffusion, 29
  Individuation, 28
  Infertility, 114
Information
  efficacy of, 86
  informed consent, 85
  procedural, 86
  sensory, 86
Intra-amniotic methods of abortion,
    146–7
Intrauterine device (coil), 116, 118

Jehovah's Witness, 117
Jews, orthodox, 112

Laparoscopy, 79
Leiden Impotence Questionnaire, 103
Lesbianism, 170, 177
Lifespan approach, 29
Life stresses
  menopause, 62, 65–6
  oestrogen levels, 65–6
  vulnerability model, 62

Male reproductive system, 92
Masculinity, 1, 2
  biological determinism, 4
  *see also* Gender
Melancholia, involutional, 61, 64